D1523166

Bird Respiration

Volume I

Editor

Timothy J. Seller
Lecturer in Zoology
Department of Pure and Applied Biology
Imperial College of Science and Technology
London

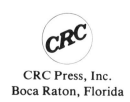

CRC Press, Inc.
Boca Raton, Florida

Library of Congress Cataloging-in-Publication Data

Bird respiration.

  Bibliography: p.
  Includes index.
  1. Birds--Physiology. 2. Respiration.
I. Seller, Timothy, J.
QL698.B544   1987   598.2'12   86-20700
ISBN-0-8493-4690-8 (Set)
ISBN-0-8493-4691-6 (v. 1)
ISBN-0-8493-4692-4 (v. 2)

Direct all inquiries to CRC Press, Inc., 2000 Corporate Blvd., N.W., Boca Raton, Florida, 33431.

© 1987 by CRC Press, Inc.

International Standard Book Number 0-8493-4690-8 (Set)
International Standard Book Number 0-8493-4691-6 (Volume I)
International Standard Book Number 0-8493-4692-4 (Volume II)

Library of Congress Card Number 86-20700
Printed in the United States

PREFACE

The earliest published work on the respiratory system of birds dates back to the middle of the seventeenth century, when Harvey described the basic structure. However, it is only in recent decades that significant advances have been made in our understanding. Earlier there was an understandable concentration of research interest on the mammalian system, and an assumption that birds must have broadly similar physiology. The two groups are comparable in a number of ways, they extend globally, occupy most types of habitat, and their respiratory systems have to provide for the requirements of evaporative cooling and vocalizations, as well as gaseous exchange. However, in at least one respect birds are superior to mammals, and this has considerable significance for the respiratory system. Birds are active at altitudes where equivalent-sized mammals would be in hypoxic collapse.[1] This functional difference is possible because of anatomical and physiological specializations of the avian system. The observed contrasts with mammals therefore are to be expected, especially since the two groups diverged at least two hundred million years ago.[2] However, the adaptations in birds are not requirements for the demanding activity of flight, since bats have typically mammalian lungs and are efficient fliers.

The anatomy of the avian air-sac and lung respiratory system and its functional consequences are covered in the chapters of this volume. However, the details are outside the authors' subject areas. A substantial literature exists on this topic, showing that there is significant interspecific variation upon the common structural plan. This is hardly suprising considering the vast range of the group, including such diverse forms as Hummingbirds, Condors, Ostriches, and Penguins. Research has taken advantage of modern technology, particularly scanning electron micrography, and the result is a detailed descriptive understanding in a number of species. The interested reader is referred to the work of A. S. King[3,4] and H.-R. Duncker,[5-8] and to the recent quantitative studies by M. A. Abdalla, J. N. Maina, and their colleagues.[9-17]

During the last two decades, a number of expansive and important reviews on avian respiration have been published. Comprehensive contributions include those by King and Molony,[18] Lasiewski,[19] Fedde,[20] Scheid,[21] and McLelland and Molony,[22] and some on specific aspects of the subject by Calder and Schmidt-Nielsen,[23] Fedde,[24] Bouverot,[25] Scheid,[26] Brackenbury,[27] and Seller and Stephenson.[28] However, all of these citations refer to papers or chapters in more general treatises on bird biology. There appears to have been only one volume dedicated to respiration, that edited by Piiper,[29] it being the proceedings of a symposium held at Göttingen, West Germany in 1977. This was a valuable contribution to the literature, but nothing similar has been published since, in spite of the large volume of research work carried out.

The present volume is intended to fill this gap and provide comprehensive reviews on the current state of research in a wide range of topics in bird respiratory physiology. It brings together a number of distinguished scientists who demonstrate the world-wide interest that exists in the subject. As editor, I am extremely grateful to those authors for their cooperation and scholarship.

T. J. Seller
May, 1986.

REFERENCES

1. **Tucker, V. A.,** Respiratory physiology of house sparrows in relation to high altitude flight, *J. Exp. Biol.,* 48, 55, 1968.
2. **Romer, A. S.,** *Vertebrate Palaeontology,* 3rd ed., University of Chicago Press, Chicago, 1966.
3. **King, A. S.,** Structural and functional aspects of the avian lungs and air sacs, *Int. Rev. Gen. Exp. Zoo.,* 2, 171, 1966.
4. **King, A. S.,** in *The Anatomy of Domestic Animals,* Vol. 2, Getty, R., Ed., Saunders, Philadelphia, 1975, 1883.
5. **Duncker, H.-R.,** The lung air sac system of birds, *Ergelm. Anat. Entwgesch.,* 45, 1, 1971.
6. **Duncker, H.-R.,** Structure of avian lungs, *Resp. Physiol.,* 14, 44, 1972.
7. **Duncker, H.-R.,** Structure of the avian respiratory tract, *Resp. Physiol.,* 22, 1, 1974.
8. **Duncker, H.-R.,** Funktionelle Anatomie des Lungen-Luftsack-Systems, in *Handbuch der Geflugelphysiologie,* Part 1, Mehner, A. and Hertfiel, W., Eds., Verlag Jena, Berlin 1983, 436.
9. **Abdalla, M. A.,** Morphometry of the avian lung, *J. Anat.,* 123, 262, 1977.
10. **Abdalla, M. A. and Maina, J. N.,** Quantitative analysis of the exchange tissue of the avian lung (Galliformes), *J. Anat.,* 133, 677, 1981.
11. **Abdalla, M. A., Main, J. N., King, A. S., King, D. Z., and Henry, J.,** Morphometrics of the avian lung. I. The domestic fowl (*Gallus gallus* variant *domesticus*), *Resp. Physiol.,* 47, 267, 1982.
12. **Maina, J. N. and King, A. S.,** Morphometrics of the avian lung. II. The wild mallard (*Anas platyrhynchos*) and graylag goose (*Anser anser*), *Resp. Physiol.,* 50, 299, 1982.
13. **Maina, J. N.,** Morphometrics of the avian lung. III. The structural design of the passerine lung, *Resp. Physiol.,* 55, 291, 1984.
14. **Maina, J. N.,** Morphometric study of the blood-gas barrier of the avian lung, *J. Anat.,* 133, 130, 1981.
15. **Maina, J. N.,** A morphometric comparison of two species of bird of different exercise capacities, *J. Anat.,* 134, 604, 1982.
16. **Maina, J. N., Abdallam, A., and King, A. S.,** Light microscopic morphometry of the lung of 19 avian species, *Acta Anat.,* 112, 264, 1982.
17. **Maina, J. N. and King, A. S.,** The thickness of the avian blood-gas barrier: qualitative and quantitative observations, *J. Anat.,* 134, 553, 1982.
18. **King, A. S. and Molony, V.,** The anatomy of respiration, in *Physiology and Biochemistry of the Domestic Fowl,* Bell, D. J. and Freeman, B., Eds., Academic Press, London, 1971, 93.
19. **Lasiewski, R. C.,** Respiratory function in birds, in *Avian Biology,* Vol. 2, Farner, D. S. and King, J. R., Eds., Academic Press, New York, 1972, 288.
20. **Fedde, M. R.,** Respiration in *Avian Physiology,* 3rd ed., Sturkie, P. D., Ed., Springer-Verlag, Berlin, 1976, 122.
21. **Scheid, P.,** Respiration and control of breathing, in *Avian Biology,* Vol. 6, Farner, D. S., King, J. R., and Parkes, K. C., Eds., Academic Press, New York, 1982, 63.
22. **McLelland, J. and Molony, V.,** Respiration in *Physiology and Biochemistry of the Domestic Fowl,* Vol. 4, Freeman, B. M., Ed., Academic Press, London, 1983, 63.
23. **Calder, W. A. and Schmidt-Nielsen,** Panting and blood carbon dioxide in birds, *Am. J. Physiol.,* 215, 417, 1970.
24. **Fedde, M. R.,** Peripheral control of avian respiration, *Fed. Proc. Fed. Am. Soc. Exp. Biol.,* 29, 1664, 1970.
25. **Bouverot, P.,** Control of breathing in birds compared with mammals, *Physiol. Rev.,* 58, 604, 1978.
26. **Scheid, P.,** Mechanisms of gas exchange in bird lungs, *Rev. Physiol. Biochem. Pharmacol.,* 86, 137, 1979.
27. **Brackenbury, J.,** Respiration and production of sounds by birds, *Biol. Rev.,* 55, 363, 1980.
28. **Seller, T. J. and Stephenson, J. D.,** Pharmacology of avian temperature regulation, in Nistico, G. and Bolis, L., Eds., *Progress in Nonmammalian Brain Research,* Vol. 2, CRC Press, Boca Raton, Fla., 1983, 105.
29. **Piiper, J., Ed.,** *Respiratory Function in Birds, Adult and Embryonic,* Springer-Verlag, Berlin, 1978, 310.

THE EDITOR

Timothy J. Seller, Ph.D., is Lecturer in Vertebrate Zoology at the Department of Pure and Applied Biology, Imperial College of Science and Technology, University of London, England.

Dr. Seller was graduated from Queen Mary College, University of London in 1967 with a B.Sc. degree in Zoology. He was awarded a Ph.D. in 1971 after research into the central neuropharmacology, centering on cholinomimetic agents, at the Institute of Psychiatry that is part of the University of London Post-Graduate Medical Federation. Since then, he has been at Imperial College, where the main theme of his research has been on the brain mechanisms of behavior. This work used bird vocalizations as a model, and has led to interests in other systems, particularly vision and respiration. His research interests range widely in birds, and include the physiology, behavior, and ecology of pest species, and, most recently, the mathematical modeling of flight. He has published over 30 papers in these areas and contributed to several books.

Dr. Seller is a regular lecturer on ornithological topics, and takes particular interest in stimulating a scientific interest in birds among the public at large.

CONTRIBUTORS

George Barnas, Ph.D.
Research Fellow
Respiratory Biology Program
Department of Environmental Science
  and Physiology
Harvard University School of Public
  Health
Boston, Massachusetts

Marvin H. Bernstein, Ph.D.
Professor
Department of Biology
New Mexico State University
Las Cruces, New Mexico

J. H. Brackenbury, Ph.D.
Sub-Department of Veterinary Anatomy
University of Cambridge
England

Nicholas John Davey, Ph.D., D.I.C.
Department of Physiology
University College London
London
England

M. Roger Fedde, Ph.D.
Professor of Physiology
Department of Anatomy and Physiology
College of Veterinary Medicine
Kansas State University
Manhattan, Kansas

Robert A. Furilla, Ph.D.
National Institutes of Health
  Postdoctoral Fellow
Department of Physiology
Dartmouth Medical School
Hanover, New Hampshire

Abbot S. Gaunt, Ph.D.
Professor
Department of Zoology
Ohio State University
Columbus, Ohio

David R. Jones, Ph.D.
Professor
Department of Zoology
University of British Columbia
Vancouver, British Columbia
Canada

Albert L. Kunz, M.D.
Professor
Department of Physiology
Ohio State University
Columbus, Ohio

Johannes Piiper, M.D.
Director
Department of Physiology
Max-Planck Institut für
  Experimentelle Medizin
Göttingen
West Germany

Werner Rautenberg, Dr. rer. nat.
Professor
Department of Biology
Ruhr-Universität
Bochum
West Germany

Peter Scheid, M.D., Ph.D.
Professor
Institut für Physiologie I
Ruhr-Universität
Bochum
West Germany

Timothy J. Seller, Ph.D.
Department of Pure and Applied
  Biology
Imperial College of Science and
  Technology
London
England

Hiroshi Tazawa, Dr. Eng., Dr. Med.
Professor
Department of Electronic Engineering
Muroran Institute of Technology
Muroran
Japan

TABLE OF CONTENTS

Volume I

Volume II

Section I: Structure and Function

Chapter 1

RESPIRATORY MUSCLES

M. Roger Fedde

TABLE OF CONTENTS

I. INTRODUCTION

Respiratory muscles are unique among skeletal muscles in being rhythmically active on a continuous basis from the time before birds hatch until they die. In this respect, they behave like cardiac muscle and possess many of the same biochemical characteristics. Unlike the myocardium, however, respiratory muscles require neural stimulation for each contraction. The rate at which they contract and the strength of that contraction, thus, is controlled by the central nervous system.

The general function of the respiratory muscles in birds is to change the volume of the combined thoracicoabdominal cavity, thereby altering pressure in the air sacs of the respiratory system with respect to that in the atmosphere. This leads to ventilation of the lungs. In contrast to most mammals, both inspiration and expiration in birds require respiratory muscular contraction, even in resting conditions.

The purpose of this chapter is to describe the structure and function of these muscles and illustrate their many interesting and unique features. Because the contractile frequency and effort of these muscles can be experimentally controlled, they provide an ideal model on which to study the mechanisms involved in producing smooth, graded contractions by skeletal muscle in general.

II. STRUCTURE OF RESPIRATORY MUSCLES

A. Gross Anatomy

Avian muscles responsible for the act of breathing are listed in Table 1. The names used in this chapter are those recently adopted by the International Committee on Avian Anatomical Nomenclature and published in the Nomina Anatomica Avium.[1] Anatomical descriptions of the respiratory muscles have been given in many books, monographs, and papers,[2-16] but the following descriptions are taken mainly from the works of deWet,[17] deWet et al.,[18] Vanden Berge,[19] and Baumel,[199] and are generally for the Chicken (*Gallus gallus*). Additional descriptions and variations in innervation can be found in Baumel[200] and Buchholz.[201]

1. Principal Respiratory Muscles

The principal respiratory muscles (Table 1) are those used during all respiratory acts, even quiet breathing. They are considered to have the most important influence on changes in celomic volume. The general position of these muscles is illustrated in the anatomical preparations shown in Figures 1 and 2 and by the drawings in Figures 3 and 4. A detailed description of the origin, insertion, and innervation of each muscle follows.

Table 1
RESPIRATORY MUSCLES IN BIRDS

Principal respiratory muscles	Accessory respiratory muscles
M. scalenus	*M. serratus superficialis*
M. costosternalis pars minor	*M. serratus profundus*
Mm. levatores costarum	*M. rhomboideus superficialis*
M. costosternalis pars major	*M. rhomboideus profundus*
Mm. intercostales interni	*M. longus colli dorsalis pars thoracica*
Mm. costoseptales	*Mm. iliocostalis et longissimus dorsi*
Mm. intercostales externi	*M. latissimus dorsi, pars cranialis et pars caudalis*
M. obliquus externus abdominis	*M. sternocoracoideus*
M. obliquus internus abdominis	
M. rectus abdominis	
M. transversus abdominis	

a. *M. scalenus* (Figures 1 through 5)

The origin of this muscle is from the transverse processes of cervical vertebrae 15 and 16. It inserts on the lateral surface of the 1st and 2nd ribs (*Costae incompletae*; these ribs do not articulate with sternal ribs and, hence, have no contact with the sternum). The *M. scalenus* has two parts: *pars cranialis* inserts on the 1st rib, and *pars caudalis* inserts on the 2nd rib. The fibers run in a caudoventral direction.

According to deWet et al.,[18] the *M. scalenus pars cranialis* of the Chicken is innervated by three to seven small branches from spinal nerves C_{15}, C_{16}, and C_{17} (Figure 5). These branches usually arise near the origin of the roots of the brachial plexus, course external to the parietal pleura, and enter the deep face of the muscle at its upper or middle third. The *M. scalenus pars caudalis* is innervated by two or three branches of the first intercostal nerve (a small branch of the ventral ramus of the 17th spinal nerve) as it courses ventrally in the first intercostal space lateral to the parietal pleura. According to Baumel,[199] the *M. scalenus* in this bird is innervated by a nerve arising from C_{13} and C_{14} and the first intercostal nerve arises from C_{16}. Variation in the organization of the brachial plexus is common in a given species and may account for these different descriptions.

b. *M. costosternalis pars minor* (Figures 1 through 6)

This small muscle originates from the dorsocaudal aspect of the *Processus craniolateralis sterni* and inserts on the distal end of the first vertebral rib and on approximately the middle third of the second vertebral rib (Figures 5 and 6). The muscle lies on the medial surface of the body wall and forms two fasciculi with fibers coursing in a dorsocaudal direction. The muscle has also been referred to as M. costisternalis pars minor and M. costisternalis pars anterior. It is innervated by branches of intercostal nerves 1 and 2.

c. *Mm. levatores costarum* (Figures 1 through 4, 6 and 7)

These muscles originate from the ventrolateral surface of the transverse processes of vertebrae C_{17}, T_1, T_2, T_3, and T_4 and insert on the cranial surface of the next caudal rib (Figures 6 and 7). They lie dorsal to the uncinate processes and tend to increase in size from caudal to cranial. The fibers run in a caudoventral direction. They are innervated by intercostal nerves 2 through 6.

d. *M. costosternalis pars major* (Figures 1 through 7)

This muscle originates from the caudal surface of the *Processus craniolateralis sterni* (Figures 6 and 7). A small slip of the muscle inserts on the distal tip of vertebral rib 2; the major part inserts on sternal ribs 3 and 4, with some fibers extending to rib 5 and only a minor insertion on rib 6. The fibers course medial to the sternal ribs in a predominantly

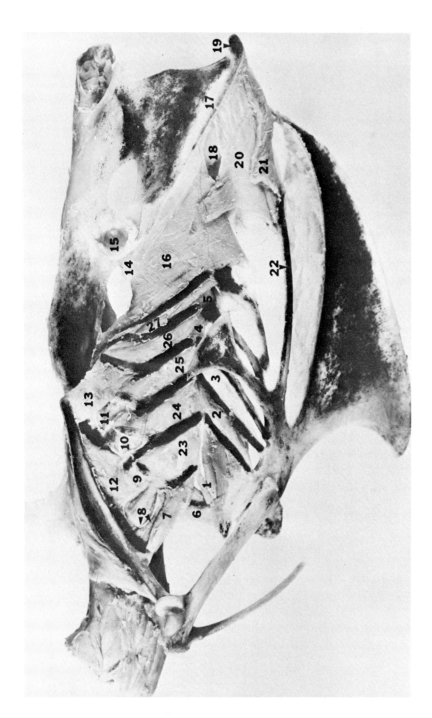

FIGURE 1.   Topographical relationships of the respiratory muscles of the Chicken, lateral view. Both the *M. rectus abdominis* and *M. obliquus externus abdominis* were partially resected to expose underlying muscles. 1 through 5, *M. costosternalis pars major*; 6, *M. costosternalis pars minor*; 7, *M. serratus superficialis pars cranialis*; 8, *M. scalenus*; 9 through 11, *Mm. levatores costarum*; 12, *M. serratus profundus*; 13, *M. serratus superficialis pars caudalis*; 14, *Tuberculum preacetabulare*; 15, *Fossa acetabuli*; 16, *M. obliquus internus abdominis*; 17, *Fenestra ischiopubica*; 18, *M. transversus abdominis*; 19, *Scapus pubis*; 20, *M. rectus abdominis*; 21, *M. obliquus externus abdominis*; 22, *Trabecula intermedia*; 23 through 27, *Mm. intercostales externi*. (From deWet, P. D., Anatomical and Physiological Investigations of the Avian Respiratory Muscles, Ph.D. thesis, University of Minnesota, Minneapolis, 1966. With permission.)

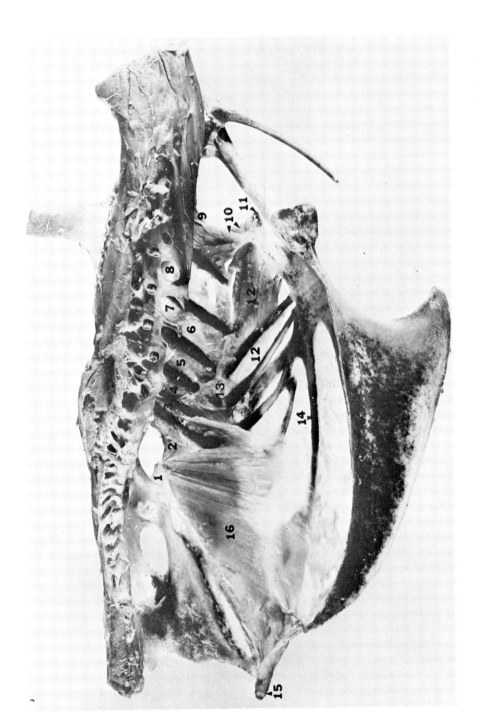

FIGURE 2. Topographical relationships of the respiratory muscles of the Chicken, medial view. 1, *Tuberculum preacetabulare*; 2, *M. obliquus internus abdominis*; 3 through 6, *Mm. intercostales interni*; 7, 8, *Mm. levatores costarum*; 9, *M. scalenus*; 10, *M. costosternalis pars minor*; 11, *Processus craniolateralis sterni*; 12, *M. costosternalis pars major*; 13, fasciculi of *Mm. costoseptales*; 14, *Trabecula intermedia*; 15, *Scapus pubis*; 16, *M. transversus abdominis*. (From deWet, P. D., Anatomical and Physiological Investigations of the Avian Respiratory Muscles, Ph.D. thesis, University of Minnesota, Minneapolis, 1966. With permission.)

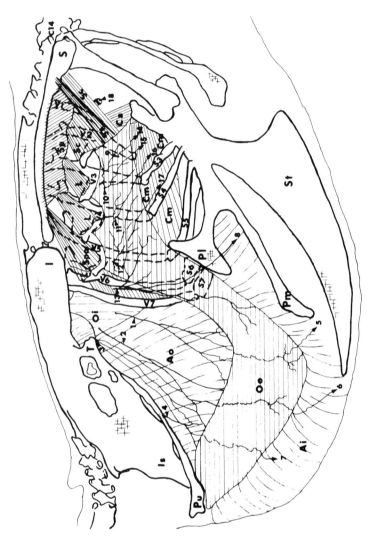

FIGURE 3.   Schematic drawing of the topographical relationships and general pattern of innervation of the respiratory muscles of the Chicken, lateral view, right side. 1, *R. lateralis ex n. lumbali 1*; 2, *R. lateralis ex n. lumbali 2 pars major*; 3, *R. lateralis ex n. lumbali 2 pars minor*; 4, *Rr. laterales ex n. lumbali 2 et 3*; 5 through 7, *Rr. cutanei laterales ex nn. lumbali 1, 2, et 3*; 8, and 14 through 17, *Rr. cutanei laterales ex nn. intercostalibus*; 9 through 13, *Nn. intercostales laterales 2, 3, 4, 5 et 6*, respectively; 18, *Plexus brachialis*; Ai, aponeurosis of insertion of *M. obliquus externus abdominis*; Ao, aponeurosis of origin of *M. obliquus externus abdominis*; C_{14}, cervical vertebra 14; Ca, *M. costosternalis pars minor*; Cm, *M. costosternalis pars major*; I, *Ilium*; Is, *Ischium*; L, *Mm. levatores costarum*; Oe, belly of *M. obliquus externus abdominis*; Oi, *M. obliquus internus abdominis*; Pl, *Trabecula lateralis*; Pm, *Trabecula intermedia*; Pu, *Scapus pubis*; S, *Scapula*; S_3 through S_7, sternal members of ribs 3 through 7, respectively; Sa, *M. serratus superficialis pars cranialis*; Sc, *M. scalenus*; Sp, *M. serratus profundus*; Spo, *M. serratus superficialis pars caudalis*; St, *Sternum*; T, *Tuberculum preacetabulare*; V_1 through V_7, vertebral member of ribs 1 through 7, respectively. The *Mm. intercostales externi* are not shown since they are covered by the *M. obliquus externus abdominis*. (From de Wet, P. D., Fedde, M. R., and Kitchell, R. L., *J. Morphol.*, 123, 17, 1967. With permission.)

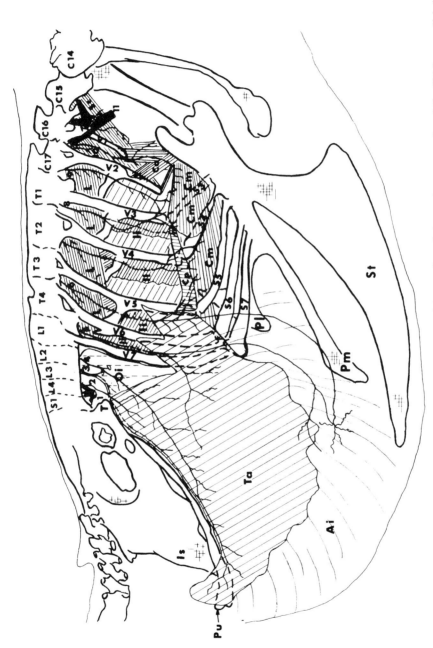

FIGURE 4. Schematic drawing of the topographical relationships and general pattern of innervation of the respiratory muscles of the Chicken, medial view, left side. 1, *Plexus lumbosacrales*; 2 through 4, *Rr. ventrales ex nn. spinalibus pars lumbalis 3, 2, et 1*, respectively; 5 through 10, *Nn. intercostales 6, 5, 4, 3, 2 et 1*, respectively; 11, *Plexus brachialis*; Ai, aponeurosis of insertion of *M. transversus abdominis*; Ca, *M. costosternalis pars minor*; Cm, *M. costosternalis pars major*; Cp, *Mm. costoseptales*; Ii, *Mm. intercostales interni*; Is, *Ischium*; L, *Mm. levatores costarum*; Oi, *M. obliquus internus abdominis*; Pl, *Trabecula lateralis*; Pm, *Trabecula intermedia*; Pu, *Scapus pubis*; S₃ through S₇, sternal members of ribs 3 through 7, respectively; Sc, *M. scalenus*; St, *Sternum*; T, *Tuberculum preacetabulare*; Ta, *M. transversus abdominis*; V₁ through V₇, vertebral member of ribs 1 through 7 respectively. (From deWet, P. D., Fedde, M. R., and Kitchell, R. L., *J. Morphol.*, 123, 17, 1967. With permission.)

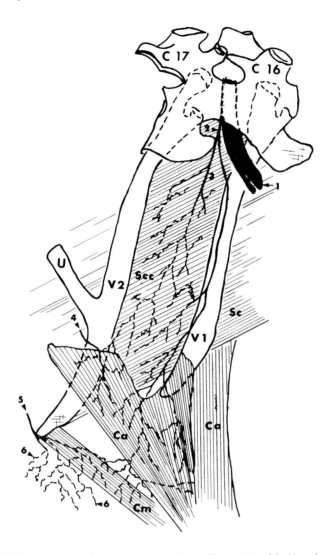

FIGURE 5. Schematic drawing of the position and innervation of the *M. scalenus pars caudalis* and *M. costosternalis pars minor* in the 1st intercostal space of the Chicken; medial view, left side. 1, *R. ventralis ex n. cervicali 17*; 2, *N. intercostalis 1*; 3, *R. muscularis ex n. intercostali 1*; 4, *R. muscularis ex n. intercostali externo 2*; 5, *R. muscularis ex n. intercostali interno 2*; 6, *Rr. musculares ad m. costosternalem partem majorem*; C_{16}, C_{17}, cervical vertebrae 16 and 17; Ca, *M. costosternalis pars minor*; Cm, *M. costosternalis pars major*; Sc, *M. scalenus pars cranialis*; Scc, *M. scalenus pars caudalis*; U, *Processus uncinatus*; V_1, V_2, vertebral members of the ribs 1 and 2. (From deWet, P. D., Fedde, M. R., and Kitchell, R. L., *J. Morphol.*, 123, 17, 1967. With permission.)

caudal direction. This muscle has been called subcostalis, triangularis sterni, transversus thoracis, and other names by earlier authors. It is innervated by terminal branches of intercostal nerves 1 through 4.

e. *Mm. intercostales interni* (Figures 2, and 4 through 7)

These muscles occur in intercostal spaces 3 through 6 in the Chicken. The fleshy belly of the muscle is replaced in the 2nd intercostal space by a membraneous connective tissue sheet (Figure 6). There is only a small fleshy belly in the cranial part of the 3rd and 4th

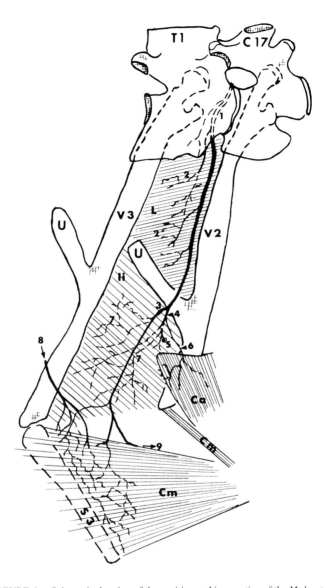

FIGURE 6.　Schematic drawing of the position and innervation of the *M. levator costae, M. intercostalis internus* (connective tissue sheet only), *M. costosternalis pars minor* and *M. costosternalis pars major* in the second intercostal space of the Chicken; medial view, left side. 1, *N. intercostalis*; 2, *Rr. musculares ad M. levatorem costae*; 3, *N. intercostalis internus*; 4, *N. intercostalis externus*; 5, *N. intercostalis lateralis*; 6, *R. muscularis ad M. costosternalem partem minorem*; 7, *Rr. musculares ad m. intercostalem externum*; 8, *R. muscularis ex n. intercostali interno 3 ad M. costosternalem partem majorem*; 9, *R. muscularis ex n. intercostali interno 2*; C_{17}, T_1, cervical vertebra 17 and thoracic vertebra 1; Ca, *M. costosternalis pars minor*; Cm, *M. costosternalis pars major*; Ii, *M. intercostalis internus* (connective tissue sheet only); L, *M. levator costae*; S_3, sternal member of rib 3; U, *Processus uncinatus*; V_2, V_3, vertebral members of ribs 2 and 3. (From deWet, P. D., Fedde, M. R., and Kitchell, R. L., *J. Morphol.*, 123, 17, 1967. With permission.)

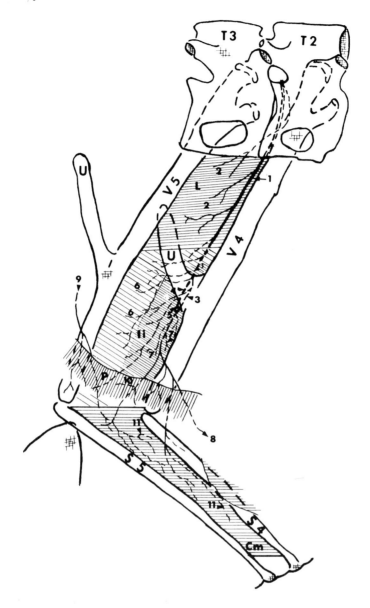

FIGURE 7.   Schematic drawing of the position and innervation of the muscles
in the 4th intercostal space of the Chicken: medial view, left side. 1, *N.
intercostalis 4*; 2, *Rr. musculares ad M. levatorem costae*; 3, *N. intercostalis
internus*; 4, *N. intercostalis externus*; 5, *N. intercostalis lateralis*; 6, *R. musculares ad n. intercostalem externum*; 7, *Rr. musculares ad M. intercostalem
internum*; 8, *R. muscularis ex n. intercostali interno 4 ad M. costosternalem
partem majorem*; 9, *R. muscularis ex n. intercostali interno 5 ad M. costosternalem partem majorem*; 10, *R. muscularis ad M. costoseptalem*; 11, *Rr.
musculares ad M. costosternalem partem majorem*; Cm, *M. costosternalis
pars major*; Ii, *M. intercostalis internus;* L, *M. levator costae*; P, *M. costo-
septalis*; S_4, S_5, sternal members of ribs 4 and 5; T_2, T_3, thoracic vertebrae 2
and 3; U, *Processus uncinatus*; V_4, V_5, vertebral members of ribs 4 and 5.
(From deWet, P. D., Fedde, M. R., and Kitchell, R. L., *J. Morphol.*, 123,
17, 1967. With permission.)

intercostal spaces, with a large caudal aponeurotic part (Figure 7); the muscle fibers occupy a large proportion of the 5th and 6th intercostal spaces. The fibers of the *Mm. intercostales interni* run from the caudal edge of a vertebral rib in a caudodorsal direction to the cranial edge of the next caudal rib, at about a 90° angle to the direction of those of the *Mm. intercostales externi*.

These muscles are innervated by the intercostal nerves in the respective intercostal spaces.

f. *Mm. costoseptales* (Figures 2, 4, and 7)

These muscles are thin, broad fasciculi (usually four in the Chicken), which originate from sternal ribs 3 through 6 at their junction with the vertebral ribs (Figure 7). They have previously been called the M. costopulmonaris and M. diaphragma. These fasciculi end in a broad aponeurosis, the horizontal septum, which has a complex insertion. It extends (1) medially over the ventral surface of the lung to the ventral processes of the thoracic vertebrae; (2) caudally to the dorsal body wall at the caudal edge of the lung; and, (3) cranially to the hilum of the lung. The entire horizontal septum has been referred to as the pulmonary diaphragm or pulmonary aponeurosis and has been described by many avian anatomists and physiologists.[20-40]

The *Mm. costoseptales* receive innervation from branches of intercostal nerves 3 through 5.

g. *Mm. intercostales externi* (Figures 1, and 5 through 7)

These muscles occur between the vertebral ribs in the 2nd through the 6th intercostal spaces. The fibers arise from the caudal surface of ribs 2 through 6 and their uncinate processes, course in a caudoventral direction, and attach on the cranial surface on the next rib caudally. The fleshy portion of each muscle is increased in size in the cranial intercostal spaces and is small in the caudal spaces. According to Zimmer,[41] the combined mass of the *Mm. intercostales externi* is larger than that of any other inspiratory muscle in the 13 species of birds that he studied. However, the mass varied widely among species ranging from 10.9% of the total respiratory muscle mass in the Vulturine Guineafowl (*Acryllium vulturinum*) to 25.0% in the Jackass Penguin (*Spheniscus demersus*).

There appears to be a relationship between the length of the uncinate process and the effectiveness of the *Mm. intercostales externi* to move the ribs. The attachment of these muscles to the ventromedial surface of uncinate processes gives them a great mechanical advantage and as they contract, the vertebral ribs are moved cranially. This, in turn, increases the angle at the junction of the vertebral and sternal ribs and increases the celomic volume. For the long uncinate processes, the muscles course almost parallel to the ribs, giving them an even greater mechanical advantage. Thus, birds with long uncinate processes and large *Mm. intercostales externi* can effect a large inspiratory effort.

The *Mm. intercostales externi* are innervated by the intercostal nerves in the respective intercostal spaces (Figures 6 and 7).

h. *M. obliquus externus abdominis* (Figures 1 and 3)

This muscle is long in the Chicken and originates from the uncinate processes and the lateral surface of the vertebral ribs as well as by an aponeurosis from the ventral border of the scapus pubis and tuberculum Preacetabulare (Figure 3). It inserts by an aponeurosis on the costal margin of the sternum, on the caudal sternal processes, and on the ventral median raphe. The muscle fibers are oriented mostly dorsoventrally over the entire course of the muscle. The innervation of this muscle is extensive, involving the intercostal nerves 2 through 6 (branches of the *N. intercostalis lateralis*) and the lateral rami of lumbar nerves 1 through 3.

i. *M. obliquus internus abdominis* **(Figures 1 through 4)**

This muscle originates by an aponeurosis from the ventral border of the pubis and the ilium (Figure 1). It inserts primarily on the caudal border of the last vertebral rib with some fibers extending downward onto the dorsal part of the sternal rib. The fibers are oriented cranioventrally at approximately a 45° angle to the synsacrum. Chinoy and George[42] divide the muscle into two parts, "anterior" and "posterior", but deWet et al.[18] contend that only the "anterior" part is the *M. obliquus internus abdominis* and the "posterior" part is actually the *M. rectus abdominis*. Chinoy and George[42] indicate that the *M. rectus abdominis* is absent in the Chicken, being replaced by a membrane, but that this muscle is present in the Pigeon (*Columba livia*). Because the origin and insertion of the "posterior" part of the muscle as described by Chinoy and George[42] appear clearly distinct from the "anterior" part and because the *M. rectus abdominis* appears to be the only muscle to develop from the distal lateral plate (somatic mesoderm) of the embryo,[43] the *M. obliquus internus abdominis* will be considered in this review to be distinct and separate from the *M. rectus abdominis*.

The *M. obliquus internus abdominis* receives its innervation from the 6th intercostal nerve (*R. muscularis ex N. intercostalis interno 6*) and from the 1st and 2nd lumbar nerves (*R. medialis ex N. lumbali 1 et 2*).

j. *M. rectus abdominis* **(Figure 1)**

The origin of this muscle is by an aponeurosis from the ventral border of the scapus pubis (Figure 1). It inserts primarily on the intermediate trabecula of the sternum. The muscle lies deep to the *M. obliquus externus abdominis* and superficial to the *M. transversus abdominis* and its fibers course in the same direction as those of the *M. obliquus internus abdominis*.

Innervation of the *M. rectus abdominis* is from the 5th and 6th intercostal nerves and the ventral rami of lumbar nerves 1 and 2.

k. *M. transversus abdominis* **(Figures 1, 2, and 4)**

This is the deepest of the abdominal muscles (Figures 2 and 4). It is a broad, flat muscle with the medial surface in contact with transversalis fascia. It originates from the medial surface of the last two or three vertebral ribs and from the ventral margin of the scapus pubis medial to the aponeurosis of origin of the *M. obliquus internus abdominis*. It inserts by an aponeurosis on the ventral median raphe and the median trabecula of the sternum. The muscle fibers run almost directly dorsoventrally. In the Chicken and the Duck (*Anas platyrhynchos*),[44] this muscle has a caudal slip that projects dorsal to the pubic bone and becomes intermingled with fibers of the *M. pubocaudalis externus* of the tail.

Innervation of the *M. transversus abdominis* comes from the 5th and 6th intercostal nerves, the 1st and 2nd lumbar nerves, and the pubic nerve (a branch of the medial femoral cutaneous nerve).

2. Accessory Respiratory Muscles

Some of these muscles may not be active during quiet breathing but are considered to aid the principal respiratory muscles during labored breathing (Table 1).

a. *M. serratus superficialis* **(Figures 1 and 3)**

There are two parts to this muscle in most birds (Figures 1). In the Chicken, the *pars cranialis* is a small muscle originating from the lateral surface of the second rib and inserting on the ventral border of the scapula near its proximal end. The *pars caudalis* originates from the lateral surface and uncinate process of vertebral rib 5 and inserts on the ventral border of the scapula at its distal end. The fibers course in a caudoventral direction. The *M. serratus superficialis pars cranialis* has been called the M. serratus ventralis cranialis and the *pars caudalis* has been termed M. serratus magnus and M. serratus ventralis caudalis in past literature.

The muscle is innervated by the superficial serratus nerve, a branch of the brachial plexus.

b. *M. serratus profundus* (Figures 1 and 3)

This muscle consists of one to several fasciculi and has been termed M. levator scapulae and M. serratus dorsalis. It originates from the caudal-most cervical vertebrae and their processes, the first few vertebral ribs, and the intervening fascia, and inserts on the medial surface of the scapula (Figure 1). It is innervated by the rhomboid and deep serratus nerves derived from the brachial plexus.

c. *M. rhomboideus superficialis*

This is a thin, flat muscle that lies just beneath the *M. latissimus dorsi, pars cranialis*, and *pars caudalis* and may consist of a pars clavicularis and pars scapularis in some species. It has been called the M. trapezius, but there is no firm evidence that the M. trapezius occurs in birds. The *M. rhomboideus superficialis* originates from the spinous processes of several cervical and thoracic vertebrae and from the pelvis. It inserts on the dorsomedial border of the scapula. The nerve supply includes the rhomboid and deep serratus nerves from the brachial plexus.

d. *M. rhomboideus profundus*

This muscle is well developed and lies deep to the *M. rhomboideus superficialis*. It originates from the spinous processes of the cervical and thoracic vertebrae, usually in common with the *M. rhomboideus superficialis*, and inserts on the dorsomedial surface of the scapula. It is innervated by the rhomboid and deep serratus nerves from the brachial plexus.

e. *M. longus colli dorsalis pars thoracica*

Others have called this the M. spinalis thoracis and M. semispinalis dorsi. It arises from the spinous processes of the movable thoracic vertebrae, median dorsal crest of the synsacrum, and the cranial border of the ilium. It inserts on several thoracic and caudal cervical vertebrae and vertebral ribs. It is innervated by dorsal rami of the thoracic nerves.

f. *Mm. iliocostalis et longissimus dorsi*

The origin of this muscle is from the craniodorsal border of the ilium and the transverse processes of several thoracic vertebrae. It inserts on the transverse processes and proximal ends of preceding vertebrae and ribs. This muscle has been separately named as M. iliocostalis and M. longissimus dorsi by previous authors. It is innervated by the dorsal branches of the thoracic spinal nerves.

g. *M. latissimus dorsi, pars cranialis et pars caudalis*

The two parts of this muscle are located just beneath the skin and constitute two distinct muscle masses in the Chicken. The *M. latissimus dorsi, pars cranialis* (often called the anterior latissimus dorsi) is a strap-like muscle arising from the spinous processes of the last few cervical and first few thoracic vertebrae. It inserts on the caudal surface of the humerus between the scapular and humeral heads of the *M. triceps brachii*. This part is darker in color than the *pars caudalis*, is a slow-contracting, tonic-type muscle with multiple innervation points on each fiber, and is extremely fatigue resistant. It can exert a continuous force on the humerus for hours without relaxation.

The *M. latissimus dorsi, pars caudalis* (often called the posterior latissimus dorsi) arises from the spinous processes of the last few thoracic vertebrae and the synsacrum, from the cranial rim of the ilium, and from adjacent ribs. It inserts by way of a flattened aponeurosis to the connective tissue sheet that surrounds the *pars cranialis*. This muscle contracts rapidly, is a twitch-type muscle, and fatigues rapidly when continuously stimulated. There is only one innervation point on each fiber.

The two parts of this muscle are unique in the animal kingdom, each being almost uniform in muscle fiber type, but one a slow-contracting muscle and the other a fast-contracting muscle. Because of this uniqueness, its structure has been studied recently to a far greater extent than that of any other avian muscle.

These muscles are innervated by the latissimus dorsi nerve from the brachial plexus.

h. *M. sternocoracoideus*

Although this muscle is included in the list of accessory respiratory muscles, its function is presently unknown and it has not been examined using electromyographic techniques. Its location may allow it to influence the sternocoracoideal articulation and thereby have a respiratory action.

The muscle is small in the Chicken and originates from the craniolateral process of the sternum. It may also arise from the sternal ribs in some birds. It inserts in the sternocoracoid impression at the base of the coracoid. It is innervated by a small branch of the supracoracoid nerve.

B. Microscopic Anatomy

The microscopic anatomy of the principal respiratory muscles has received relatively little attention. On the other hand, the microstructure of the accessory respiratory muscle, the *M. latissimus dorsi, pars cranialis et pars caudalis*, has been extensively studied.[15,45-80] The following discussion will, however, be devoted mainly to those muscles known to be involved with eupneic breathing.

1. Histochemical Fiber Types

Using the nomenclature proposed by Peter el al.,[81] three types of muscle fibers can be recognized in most mammalian and avian muscles using histochemical techniques. The first type, fast-twitch-glycolytic fibers (FG), has high activity of myofibrillar adenosine triphosphatase (ATPase) and stains darkly when preincubated at pH 10.3, indicating rapid contraction capability. These fibers also have high activity of phosphorylase (Pase), indicating high activity of glycolytic enzymes. These fibers have low activity of reduced nicotinamide adenine dinucleotide diaphorase (NADDase), indicating poor capability to generate ATP through oxidative reactions, and stain lightly for this enzyme. These fibers can contract rapidly but they fatigue quickly. The second type, slow-twitch-oxidative fibers (SO), stains lightly for myofibrillar ATPase, indicating slow contraction, but stains intermediately to darkly for reduced NADDase activity, indicating high ability to generate ATP from oxidative reactions. These muscle fibers contract more slowly than FG fibers, but are resistant to fatigue and capable of prolonged contraction. The third type, fast-twitch-oxidative-glycolytic fibers (FOG), stains with either a high or intermediate intensity for myofibrilliar ATPase activity, but also stains intensely for reduced NADDase activity. These fibers can contract rapidly and are fatigue resistant. These three types of fibers are also termed "fast-twitch, fatigable (FF)", "slow-twitch, fatigue resistant (SR)", and "fast-twitch, fatigue resistant (FR)", respectively, in accordance with their functional properties.[82-84] Other classification schemes have been proposed for avian muscle.[58,85]

The histochemical characteristics of many of the principal respiratory muscles of the Pigeon and Chicken have been described.[15,42,86,87] All of these muscles contain a mixture of fibers with respect to both enzyme activities and size. However, there are substantial quantitative differences among these muscles (Figures 8 and 9). In some muscles, those

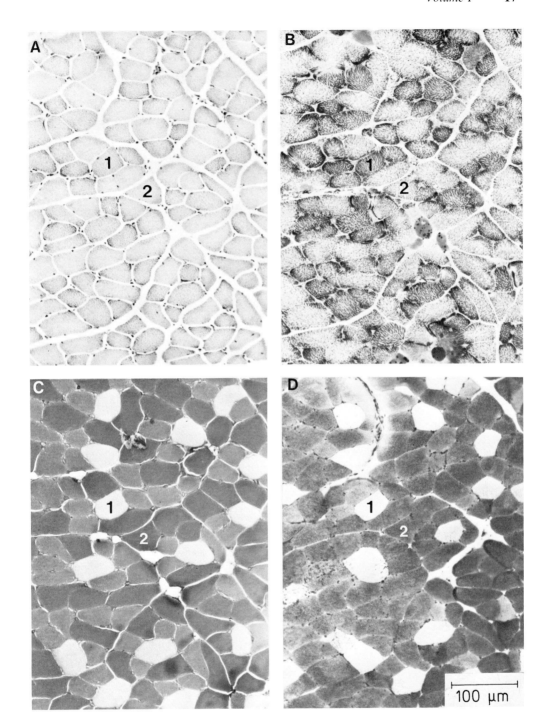

FIGURE 8. Adjacent sections illustrating the histological and histochemical features of the *Mm. costoseptales* of the adult Chicken. Note that the fiber diameter of all fiber types is small. (A) Hematoxylin-eosin stain; (B) nicotinamide adenine dinucleotide diaphorase activity; (C) myofibrillar adenosine triphosphatase activity (preincubation pH 10.3); (D) phosphorylase activity. The same two fibers are numbered in each picture.

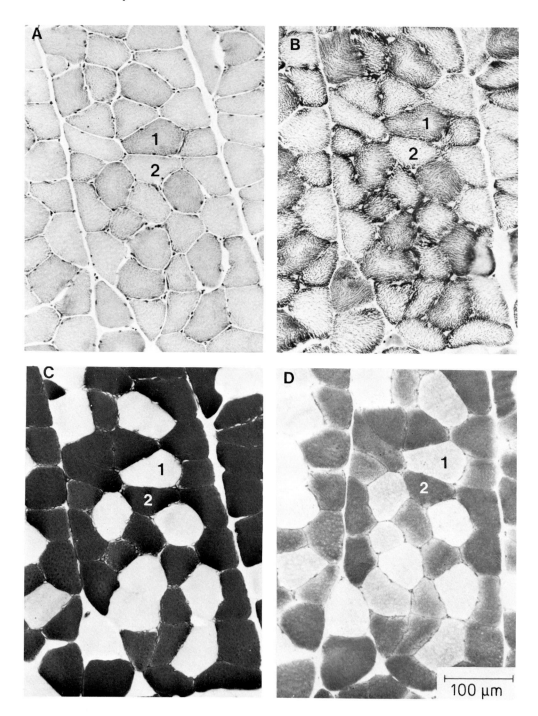

FIGURE 9.   Adjacent sections illustrating histological and histochemical features of the *M. costosternalis pars major* of the adult Chicken. Fiber diameters are among the largest for respiratory muscles in this bird. (A) Hematoxylin-eosin stain; (B) nicotinamide adenine dinucleotide diaphorase activity; (C) myofibrillar adenosine triphosphatase activity (preincubation pH 10.3); (D) phosphorylase activity. The same two fibers are numbered in each picture.

Table 2
PROPORTION OF MYOFIBERS STAINING DARK AND LIGHT
FOR MYOFIBRILLAR ATPase[a] ACTIVITY IN VARIOUS
RESPIRATORY MUSCLES OF THE CHICKEN

Muscle	High myofibrillar ATPase activity		Low myofibrillar ATPase activity	
	%	Cross-sectional area (μm^2)	%	Cross-sectional area (μm^2)
M. costosternalis pars major	68	3631	32	4072
M. costosternalis pars minor	72	3848	28	4072
Mm. intercostales externi	73	4185	27	3959
Mm. intercostales interni	77	3632	23	4301
M. obliquus internus abdominis	83	4300	17	2734
M. scalenus	83	3632	17	3526
M. transversus abdominis	88	2469	12	1963
Mm. costoseptales	89	1662	11	1452
M. obliquus externus abdominis	90	2642	10	2290
M. rectus abdominis	90	2986	10	1662

[a]   Preincubation at pH 10.3.

Data from Fedde and Cardinet[87] and Fedde et al.[182]

fibers staining darkly for myofibrillar ATPase activity are larger than those staining lightly, whereas in others, the situation is reversed (Table 2). In addition, a fourth histochemical fiber type appears to be present in most respiratory muscles of the Chicken, although in small numbers (5% or less of the total fiber population) (Table 3). This fiber type has low activities for all three enzymes, myofibrillar ATPase, NADDase, and Pase, and, therefore, can be considered to be slow-contracting as well as rapidly fatigable (SF).

As might be expected in muscles that are active for a large fraction of the animal's life, most fibers in respiratory muscles of the Chicken have the capability to contract rapidly with low susceptibility to fatigue (Table 3). However, the *M. obliquus externus abdominis* is an exception in that most of its fibers appear to be rapidly fatigable. The respiratory muscles also vary in the fraction of slow-contracting fibers from a high of over 25% in the *M. costosternalis pars minor* to a low of about 8% in the *M. rectus abdominis*. Thus, the various fibers in respiratory muscles possess several combinations of myofibrillar ATPase, NADDase, and Pase activities, providing the range of functional characteristics necessary for cyclic activity with resistance to fatigue required for respiration, and intermittent, fast contractions to generate the large tensions required for vocalization, coughing, and other nonrespiratory activities.

2. Muscle Fiber Uniformity

Measurements of muscle fiber diameter and cytochemical characteristics usually are based on samples taken from only a single, or at most few, sites along a muscle length. For these measurements to be useful in estimating the fraction of each fiber type within the muscle as a whole, one must be certain that those characteristics are constant along the length of each single fiber.

To determine if fibers in the *M. transversus abdominis* of the Chicken are uniform throughout their length, the same muscle fibers have been identified and characterized histochemically at 10 to 20 locations along their entire course.[86] Although small fluctuations in diameter occurred along the length of a fiber in this muscle, fibers retained their relative

Table 3
PROPORTION OF MUSCLE FIBERS WITH VARIOUS FUNCTIONAL CHARACTERISTICS IN RESPIRATORY MUSCLES OF THE CHICKEN

Muscle	Functional characteristics			
	FR (%)[a]	FF (%)[b]	SR (%)[c]	SF (%)[d]
M. costosternalis pars major	38.8	32.5	25.5	3.2
M. costosternalis pars minor	49.7	24.1	25.2	1.0
Mm. intercostales externi	48.4	24.3	25.0	2.3
Mm. intercostales interni	48.9	25.1	20.7	5.3
Mm. obliquus internus abdominis	55.6	27.1	15.9	1.4
Mm. costoseptales	62.1	27.8	8.3	1.8
M. obliquus externus abdominis	18.6	71.4	8.9	1.1
M. rectus abdominis	46.5	45.3	8.2	0

[a] FR = fast contracting-fatigue resistant.
[b] FF = fast contracting-fatigable.
[c] SR = slow contracting-fatigue resistant.
[d] SF = slow contracting-fatigable.

Data from Fedde and Cardinet.[87]

size (large, intermediate, or small) throughout their length. Likewise, NADDase and my-ofibrillar ATPase activities were either consistently high or low in a given fiber at all points along its length. Thus, it appears that muscle fibers are homogeneous in their size and histochemical characteristics, as might be expected if these properties are in some way controlled by a trophic factor from the innervating neuron.[88]

3. Muscle Spindles

Muscle spindles are complex, encapsulated sense organs possessing one or more modified muscle fibers (called intrafusal fibers) and several types of innervation. They are currently thought to sense voluntary movement and assess deviations from that movement.[89] They also may be involved in kinesthesia, the perception of changes in the angles of joints.

The presence of avian muscle spindles was described many years ago,[90-92] but their structural details have been elucidated only recently. The lastest studies have focused on: (1) the number of spindles in various muscles, number of intrafusal fibers per spindle, size of the spindle, and position of spindles within a muscle;[93-104] (2) the division of the intrafusal fibers into various types based on fiber size and number of nuclei in the equatorial region,[94,97,99,102,105] on histochemical activities of various enzymes,[67,74,104,106-110] or on ultrastructural characteristics;[111-114] (3) the structure of the spindle capsule and connective tissue surrounding the intrafusal fibers;[69,93,94,99,105] (4) the afferent and efferent innervation of the intrafusal fibers;[93,94,102,105,109,111,115-117] (5) the blood supply to the spindles;[112,118] and (6) the development of spindles during the following embryonic life.[109,110]

a. Presence in Respiratory Muscles

Despite the large number of studies on morphology of spindles in avian muscles, only one study has examined them in a respiratory muscle.[119] Previous to that study, a continuous efferent discharge of small-amplitude impulses had been found in the nerves to the *M. transversus abdominis* in the Chicken when apnea was induced by lowering the intrapulmonary CO_2 concentration (see Section III.B). Similar observations in nerves to the *M. intercostales* of the cat by Sears[120] had been interpreted as being due to the tonic activity of gamma efferent fibers that provide motor innervation to muscle spindles. Therefore, it was anticipated that the *M. transversus abdominis* would have an abundance of muscle spindles. However, when this muscle was serially sectioned and examined at 90-μm intervals in six Chickens, no spindles were found in four birds, only one spindle in one bird, and five spindles in the other bird.[119] Thus, this muscle is similar to the extraocular muscles of the Japanese Quail (*Coturnix coturnix japonica*), Pigeon, Sparrow (*Passer domesticus*), Canary (*Serinus canaria*),[95] and the caudal belly of the biventer cervicus muscle of the Chicken[93] in having few or no muscle spindles. Hence, an alternative interpretation of the function of the efferent nerve impulses to this muscle during apnea must be put forth (see Section III.B.1).

b. Structural Characteristics

Those muscle spindles found in the *M. transversus abdominis* of the Chicken exhibited similar morphological features to spindles located in other avian muscles.[97,102] The spindle length ranged from 890 to 4680 μm with equatorial diameters ranging from 55 to 138 μm; there were two to six intrafusal fibers in each spindle. One spindle, serially reconstructed by examining each serial section (6 μm thick) throughout about two thirds of its length, is illustrated in Figure 10. This spindle had four intrafusal fibers in the equatorial region, one of which branched in the juxtaequatorial region, a common finding in mammalian spindles.[121] The intrafusal fibers were all of similar length. In addition, the spindle capsule did not enclose the ends of the spindle but became thickened into several layers in the equatorial zone. There was also a dense layer of connective tissue around each intrafusal fiber in this region.

Like spindles in other avian muscles, the intrafusal fibers in spindles in the *M. transversus abdominis* did not possess large accumulations of nuclei in the equatorial region and, therefore, did not resemble nuclear bag fibers in mammalian spindles. Nuclei were present in rows in all fibers, similar to those found in mammalian nuclear chain fibers. Although histochemical techniques were not applied to the spindles examined in the *M. transversus abdominis*, two general degrees of myofibrillar density were found in the intrafusal fibers (Figure 10). In some areas, the myofibrillae were densely packed and no definite fields of Cohnheim were present, while in other areas the myofibrillae were widely spread and fields of Cohnheim were readily apparent. Thus, the myofibrillar density was not constant throughout the length of the intrafusal fibers. This contrasts with the uniform histochemical features of the extrafusal fibers (as discussed in Section II.B.2), and with the similarity of histochemical reactions over short lengths of intrafusal fibers in spindles from the *M. flexor carpi ulnaris* of the Pigeon.[108]

Three types of intrafusal fibers in avian muscle spindles have been delineated using the electron microscope.[113] One type has tightly packed myofilaments without M bands in the middle of the sarcomere, a second type has tightly packed myofilaments but with M bands, and a third type has large spaces between myofilaments with M bands always present. Three fiber types also have been described using histochemical techniques.[107]

Although many nerve fibers were found in the equatorial region of muscle spindles from the *M. transversus abdominis*, they were not observed to form an annulospiral ending around the intrafusal fibers. Investigations of the innervation of avian muscle spindles from nonrespiratory muscles with the electron microscope also demonstrate differences in the sensory endings, as compared to mammalian spindles.[117]

4. Capillary Blood Supply to Various Fiber Types

It has been well demonstrated that the blood capillary density (capillaries per square millimeter of muscle) is considerably higher for mammalian muscles containing fibers with high oxidative enzyme activities than for muscles containing fibers with low activities.[122]

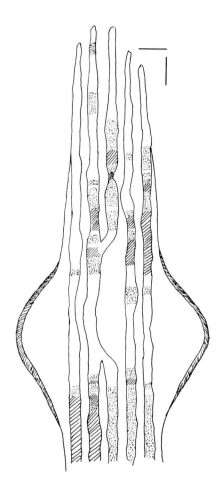

FIGURE 10.   Schematic drawing of a muscle spindle from the *M. transversus abdominis* in the Chicken. Four intrafusal fibers are present, one of which branched on each side of the equatorial region. Different histological features of the intrafusal fibers are represented by stippling (areas with a moderate degree of myofibrillar spacing and apparent fields of Cohnheim), cross-hatching (areas with extreme degrees of myofibrillar spacing and prominent fields of Cohnheim), and clear areas (compact myofibrillar arrangement with no definite fields of Cohnheim). The clear areas in the equatorial region are undefined because myofibrillar spacing is not clear. Horizontal bar represents 20 μm and is the scale for spindle width; vertical bar represents 165 μm and is the scale for spindle length. (From deWet, P. D., Farrell, P. R., and Fedde, M. R., *Poult. Sci.*, 50, 1349, 1971. With permission.)

This seems logical, since the vascularity of tissues should be related to the O_2 requirements.[123] These observations have been extended using electron-microscopic techniques to directly examine mitochondrial density.[124] However, substantial variability occurs in the number of capillaries per unit volume of muscle fibers containing the same mitochondrial density; thus, physiological factors such as blood flow, perfusion distribution, and O_2 diffusion facilitation have been proposed to more fully account for the relationship between the vascular supply to a muscle fiber and its metabolic activities.

Extensions of these studies have been applied to avian muscles. The avian muscles most studied from anatomical, physiological,[52,55,70,78,79,125-145] and biochemical[146-160] standpoints have been the *M. latissimus dorsi, pars cranialis* and *pars caudalis*, which, as indicated in Table 1, may be considered accessory respiratory muscles. The highly oxidative *M. latissimus dorsi, pars cranialis* of the chicken has 24% more capillaries per fiber and 25% more capillaries per square millimeter than the *M. latissimus dorsi, pars caudalis*. In addition, the former muscle has 29% of its capillaries open to blood flow at any one time during rest, compared to only 11% in the latter muscle.[80] However, the capillary configuration is quite different between these two muscles; numerous intercapillary anastomoses allow a circuitous route for blood flow from arteriole to venuole in the *M. latissimus dorsi, pars cranialis*, whereas in the *M. latissimus dorsi, pars caudalis* there is a simple, parallel arrangement of capillaries with little intercapillary connection.[145] Functional studies indicate that blood flow through these two muscles is similar, despite differences in the metabolic properties of their muscle fibers.[145]

Capillary blood flow through both *Mm. latissimus dorsi, pars cranialis* and *pars caudalis* may be controlled by the local concentration of adenosine in the extracellular space surrounding the resistance vessels. When the blood flow to either resting muscle is briefly stopped, there is no great change in creatine phosphate or adenosine nucleotide content, but adenosine concentration markedly increases.[159] In addition, reactive hyperemia is similar in both muscles following blood flow occlusions in concert with similar concentrations of adenosine.[141] Hence, the mechanisms utilized to control blood flow in both muscles appear similar.

Studies of the structural or functional capillary blood supply to the various fiber types in the primary avian respiratory muscles have not been conducted, although total blood flow to the *M. transversus abdominis* in both Pekin Ducks and Bar-Headed Geese (*Anser indicus*) increases when these muscles increase their tension during hyperpnea induced by hypoxia.[161] Because of the continuous use of the primary respiratory muscles and because of the high oxidative characteristics of many of their fibers but low oxidative characteristics of others, they may provide an ideal model on which to study the relationship of capillary supply to metabolic requirement.

III. FUNCTION OF RESPIRATORY MUSCLES

A. Action during Breathing

1. Phases of the Respiratory Cycle When Muscles Are Active

Early investigators attempted to determine if various respiratory muscles contracted during inspiration or expiration in birds by visual inspection, by recording of sternal movements, and by anatomical considerations of origins and insertions.[29,162-166] Physical models also have been useful to illustrate the importance of the uncinate processes and the muscles that insert on them in the process of breathing.[41] However, the unequivocal solution to this problem for many of the muscles had to await the use of electromyographic recording techniques. By recording the electrical activity of muscles, it was possible to state not only during which phase of the respiratory cycle the activity occurred, but also exactly when during the cycle the muscles began and ceased their activity.[38,167-172]

The phase of the respiratory cycle when the principal and accessory respiratory muscles are active is indicated in Table 4. As can be seen in this table, the action of the *Mm. intercostales* is complex. Most of the *Mm. intercostales externi* are active during inspiration but those muscles in the 5th and 6th intercostal spaces are active during expiration; most of the *Mm. intercostales interni* are active during expiration; but that in the 2nd intercostal space is active during inspiration. According to deWet et al.,[18] both *Mm. intercostalis interni* and *externi* are absent in the 1st intercostal space in the Chicken.

Table 4
ACTION OF THE PRINCIPAL AND ACCESSORY RESPIRATORY MUSCLES OF THE CHICKEN

Inspiratory	Expiratory
M. scalenus	*Mm. intercostales externi* of 5th and 6th spaces
Mm. intercostales externi (except in 5th and 6th spaces)	*Mm. intercostales interni* of 3rd to 6th spaces
M. intercostalis interni in 2nd space	*M. costosternalis pars minor*
M. costosternalis pars major	*M. obliquus externus abdominis*
Mm. levatores costarum	*M. obliquus internus abdominis*
M. serratus profundus	*M. transversus abdominis*
	M. rectus abdominis
	M. serratus superficialis pars cranialis et caudalis
	Mm. costoseptales
	M. rhomboideus superficialis
	M. rhomboideus profundus
	M. latissimus dorsi
	Mm. iliocostalis et longissimus dorsi
	M. longus colli dorsalis pars thoracica

All of the abdominal muscles are expiratory in function. Additional muscles in the dorsal region of the thorax (*M. rhomboideus superficialis, M. latissimus dorsi, M. rhomboideus profundus, Mm. iliocostalis et longissimus dorsi*, and *M. longus colli dorsalis pars thoracica*), exhibit electrical activity that is not always related to a particular phase of the respiratory cycle during quiet breathing; however, in many cases, these muscles are electrically active during expiration.[168,169] The *M. pectoralis, M. supracoracoideus*, or *M. subscapularis* do not exhibit electrical potentials related to resting respiratory movement.

Special mention should be made of the function of the *Mm. costoseptales* and their action on the pulmonary aponeurosis. As early as 1896, Soum[29] stated that these muscles contracted during expiration and had the function of producing tension on the aponeurosis, thus preventing collapse of the air sac ostia and bronchial orifices, which penetrated this structure. He postulated that the tension of this aponeurosis remained essentially constant throughout the respiratory cycle by action of these muscles during expiration and by passively being pulled by the separation of the ribs during inspiration. Recent estimates of the force applied to the aponeurosis by increased air-sac pressures and the maximal force capable of being generated by the *Mm. costoseptales* in the Ostrich (*Struthio camelus*) suggest that approximately 300 times more force can be generated by the muscles than is required to prevent distortion during quiet breathing.[173] Thus, although there are small volume changes (1.4%) of the avian lung during breathing,[173] these muscles may act as predicted by Soum[29] to minimize lung-volume changes and prevent occlusion of bronchial structures during expiration.

2. Influence of Bodily Position

It has long been recognized that respiratory movements of birds are markedly changed when they are placed in the unnatural supine position.[41] The tidal volume may be reduced by as much as one half when unanesthetized Chickens are placed on their backs.[174] In addition, the vertical displacement of the sternum at its apex is about twice as great in Chickens placed in the supine compared with the upright position.[175] These larger sternal movements coincided with a higher respiratory frequency and a larger end-expiratory carbon dioxide concentration. Thus, it is to be expected that the respiratory muscles are contracting with greater force in the supine position but that the higher resistance to gas flow in the respiratory system causes a reduced parabronchial ventilation. However, as found by Fedde et al.,[171] no consistent difference in the electromyograms of either inspiratory or expiratory muscles could be detected when the birds were changed from the upright to the supine position.[175] Possibly, problems of maintaining the electrodes in exactly the same position in the muscle during the repositioning process masked any electrical change that actually occurred.

When birds are in the totally relaxed state, the sternum is in a midposition between its maximum at the end of inspiration and at the end of expiration. The action of both inspiratory and expiratory muscles deforms the thoracic cage, thereby imparting energy to the tissues of that structure. That energy can be used to aid the first half of each phase of the respiratory cycle. Thus, at the end of expiration in the upright bird, the sternum is aided in moving toward its midposition by the elastic recoil of the thoracic cage and by the gravitational action on the mass of the pectoral muscles and viscera resting on the inner surface of the sternum. At the peak of inspiration, the elastic recoil of the thoracic cage is the only passive force acting to move the sternum to its midposition and that action is counteracted by the gravitational pull on the pectoral mass and viscera. When a Chicken is placed on its back, the time required for the sternum to reach its midposition from the peak of expiration is markedly increased,[171] illustrating the influence of the force of gravity on the pectoral muscle mass and viscera.

Although Soum[29] proposed that the elastic recoil of the thoracic cage was mainly responsible for the initial movements of both phases of the respiratory cycle, electromyographic recordings have demonstrated that the muscles of respiration are also active at this time (Figure 11). The inspiratory muscles become active only a few milliseconds after the initiation of an inspiratory sternal movement and their activity does not cease completely until well after the beginning of expiration. The expiratory muscles become active even before the sternum begins its expiratory movement and remain active for some time into the inspiratory cycle. Thus, the smooth transition between expiration and inspiration appears to result because of opposing tensions brought about by activity of both sets of muscles.

3. Effects of Anesthesia

Most general anesthetics depress the central respiratory neuronal pool at the same time that higher centers are depressed.[176] These drugs inhibit activation of large motoneurons to respiratory muscles and decrease the frequency of discharge in smaller motoneurons as well.[171] An increase in the initial rate of sternal movement during both phases of the respiratory cycle has been reported in the Chicken, presumably because of a reduced antagonism of opposing muscular groups to the inherent elastic recoil of the stretched thoracic cage. Deep anesthesia generally results in lowered tidal volume and altered blood gas tensions for O_2 and CO_2 as a result of the depressed ventilation.

4. Effects of Bilateral Vagotomy

Bilateral vagotomy alters the pattern of breathing, principally by prolonging expiration and increasing the amplitude of the breath.[177-179] Electromyographic recordings from a variety of inspiratory and expiratory muscles show that the muscles are active throughout their respective respiratory cycles after vagotomy, including the prolonged expiratory phase.[172] The expiratory muscles remain active for a longer time after the beginning of the inspiratory sternal movement following section of these nerves, suggesting that this phase of the cycle is not as abruptly halted as in the normal condition. Hence, the central respiratory neuronal pool remains active after vagotomy, but the switching mechanism responsible for changing phases is markedly disrupted.

B. Motor-Unit Recruitment Pattern

The motor unit may be considered the functional unit of the neuromuscular system. It is defined as the motoneuron and all of the muscle fibers that it innervates. The term "muscle unit" is given to those muscle fibers in a motor unit.

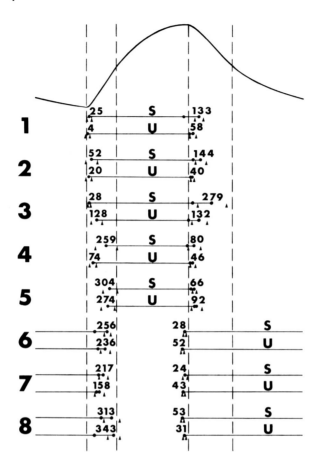

FIGURE 11.   Timing of respiratory muscle activity in relation to movement of the sternum in anesthetized Chickens in the upright (U) and supine (S) positions. Electromyograms were recorded from muscles on the right side of the birds. The smooth curve at the top represents a complete respiratory cycle with inspiration directed upward and expiration directed downward. The dashed vertical lines indicate from left to right: beginning of inspiration, resting position of the sternum, beginning of expiration, resting position of the sternum. The muscles studied are numbered on the left: 1, *M. scalenus*; 2, *M. costosternalis pars major*; 3, through 7, *M. intercostalis externis* in the 2nd through 6th intercostal spaces, respectively; 8, *M. obliquus internus abdominis*. The horizontal bars indicate the average period of electrical activity for the various muscles. The numbers indicate the time in milliseconds after or before the beginning of inspiration (on the left) or expiration (in the center of the figure). At the end of each bar, two dots are shown. The first dot indicates the time when approximately 80% of the peak electrical activity of the muscle had ceased, whereas the end dot indicates when the electrical activity was reduced to base-line noise. The number is associated with the latter dot. The triangles indicate the range of the standard error of the means represented by the dots at the ends of the bars. (From Fedde, M. R., Burger, R. E., and Kitchell, R. L., *Poult. Sci.*, 43, 839, 1964. With permission.)

1. Orderly Motor-Unit Recruitment

Voluntary contraction of a skeletal muscle is a very orderly process. An individual motor unit begins to discharge at a precisely defined stage of the contraction and increases its discharge frequency as contraction increases. Sequentially, other motor units begin to discharge as more tension generation occurs. Such a pattern of motor-unit recruitment has been extensively described in many mammalian limb muscles and an underlying principle has emerged that the size of the motoneuron determines its susceptibility to recruitment.[180]

The small motoneurons are the first to be activated, followed successively by larger and larger motoneurons. Small motoneurons are the most abundant neurons innervating skeletal muscle. They have small axons and innervate relatively few muscle fibers. Small motoneurons are the easiest to recruit because they have a high input resistance and, thus, a large excitatory postsynaptic potential is generated across their dendritic membrane when stimulated by activity of impinging synaptic endings. For this reason, fewer active synaptic endings from other neurons are required to produce a threshold-level depolarization at the axon hillock of the small motoneurons and cause impulse discharge. The large motoneurons, on the other hand, have a low input resistance because of their large cell-surface area, and many more simultaneously activated synaptic endings on their dendritic membranes are required to produce an excitatory postsynaptic potential large enough to cause these motoneurons to discharge an impulse at their axon hillock. Large motoneurons are brought into activity only when tension demands are high in voluntary muscle contraction.

The motoneuronal recruitment pattern in respiratory muscles of birds follows the identical plan described above for mammalian muscles. That pattern was noted in the earliest study on birds using electromyographic techniques in which Loofbourrow and Gesell[181] noted: "In the chicken both inspiratory and expiratory contractions show the slowly augmenting inspiratory pattern of activity characteristic for the inspiratory muscles of the dog, mouse, rat, rabbit, and horse. Frequency of muscle fiber twitch and recruitment of newly activated units were found to increase with the progress of each act." The slowly augmenting discharge pattern of muscle units was clearly evident in the majority of single muscle-unit recordings from either inspiratory or expiratory muscles shown by Kadono and Okada[168] and Kadono et al.[169] The muscle-unit discharge began slowly and increased in frequency as contraction continued, usually reaching a maximum at or near the peak of contraction.

The orderly recruitment of motor units during various strengths of contraction of the *M. transversus abdominis* has been studied in the Chicken during unidirectional ventilation.[182] Using that technique, all degrees of muscle tension from that at apnea to that during dyspnea can be induced in a completely physiological manner by changing the concentration of carbon dioxide in the ventilating gas stream from low levels to higher levels (Figure 12). With low intrapulmonary CO_2 concentrations, apnea occurs. However, there is still a tonic motoneuronal discharge by small neurons that produces small motor-unit potentials in the muscle (not shown in Figure 12). This activity results in a small amount of maintained tension (Figure 13). Similar small potentials in motor nerves to the intercostal muscles of the cat have been thought to be due to active gamma efferent neurons to the intrafusal fibers of muscle spindles.[120,183] However, as is seen in Section II.B.3, the *M. transversus abdominis* has few or no muscle spindles. Furthermore, activity of muscle spindles could not account for the uniform distribution of electromyographic activity in the muscle nor the tension produced by it during apnea. Thus, in the Chicken, small motoneurons innervating a small number of muscle fibers appear capable of producing a small degree of continuous muscle contraction, a feature that could be important not only for the process of breathing but also for providing an appropriate degree of compliance to the abdominal wall.

As the *M. transversus abdominis* begins to contract in a rhythmic manner, there is recruitment of progressively larger and larger motoneurons, each of which innervates larger muscle units. The muscle units, in turn, generate larger motor-unit potentials and produce larger tensions (Figure 12). In addition, the electrical activity of the expiratory motoneurons becomes completely inhibited during at least a major portion of the inspiratory phase of the respiratory cycle. Thus, even the small motoneurons, which are easiest to recruit, can be completely inhibited when activity in the opposing muscle group is high.

The motor-unit recruitment pattern seen in the *M. transversus abdominis* of the anesthetized adult Chicken is also present in the day-old Chick[184] where the histochemical differentiation of the fiber types has not occurred.[17] Thus, the organization of motoneuronal excitability is

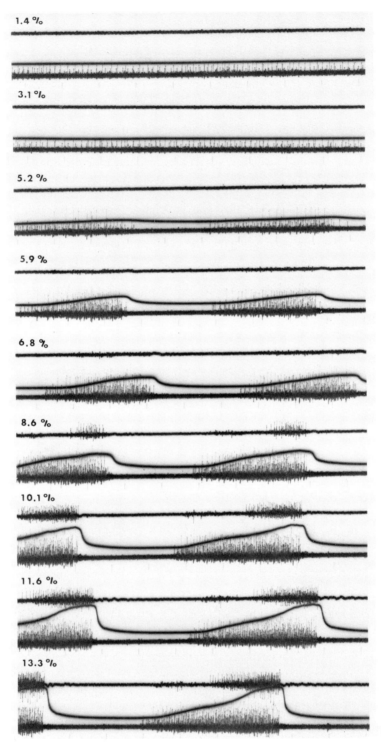

FIGURE 12.   Pattern of motor-unit recruitment during various strengths of contraction in the *M. transversus abdominis* of the anesthetized Chicken. Each set of three tracings was taken at the intrapulmonary CO_2 concentration (ranging from 1.4 to 13.3%) indicated on the left. For each set of tracings, the top trace shows the electromyographic activity in the muscle; the middle trace shows the sternal movement, expiration up, inspiration down; the bottom trace shows the efferent electrical activity in a small nerve branch to the muscle. The time marks at the bottom of each set of tracings occur every 0.5 sec. (From Fedde, M. R., deWet, P. D., and Kitchell, R. L., *J. Neurophysiol.*, 32, 995, 1969. With permission.)

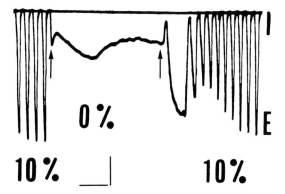

FIGURE 13. Tonic tension produced by the *M. transversus abdominis* of the anesthetized Chicken during apnea. Top line indicates the minimal tension at the peak of inspiration with 10% CO_2 in the unidirectional gas stream ventilating the lungs. The CO_2 was suddenly removed from the gas stream at the first arrow and the bird immediately went into apnea. However, a small amount of tonic tension remained. CO_2 was returned to the ventilating gas stream at the second arrow and phasic contractions returned. I, inspiration; E, expiration. Vertical scale, 20 g; horizontal scale, 10 sec. (From Fedde, M. R., deWet, P. D., and Kitchell, R. L., *J. Neurophysiol.*, 32, 995, 1969. With permission.)

developed before the muscle is biochemically heterogeneous. The histochemical characteristics of the developing fibers may be determined, at least in part, by the activity pattern in the motoneurons innervating them. In addition, a similar motor-unit recruitment pattern occurs in unanesthetized, adult Chickens.[185] The suppression of the central nervous system by an anesthetic does not appear to selectively affect one motoneuron population, but instead, lowers the degree of excitability of all neurons making the larger motoneurons very difficult to recruit.[177]

2. Histochemical Features of Muscle-Units in Relation to Recruitment Pattern

The motor-unit recruitment pattern in the adult bird described above is likely to be related to the histochemical pattern of the muscle units in the respiratory muscles.[182] A small fraction of the muscle fibers have low activities of myofibrillar ATPase but high activities of enzymes involved in ATP production by aerobic pathways. These fibers might be expected to be innervated by motoneurons that are recruited easily and capable of providing almost constant tension without fatigue. A larger fraction of the fibers have a higher myofibrillar ATPase activity but also a high activity of enzymes involved in aerobic metabolism; these fibers could provide rapid contractions but also be capable of sustained contraction with little fatigue. Over half of the fibers have high activities of myofibrillar ATPase but lower activities of the aerobic enzymes and might be expected to be recruited into activity only when tension demands are great, and then only for short periods of time. Although direct evidence for such a relationship among motoneurons, muscle fiber types, and contraction tensions is not available for birds, such a situation does exist in mammalian muscles.[83,84]

C. Action during Nonrespiratory Activities

The respiratory muscles, especially those involved with expiration, provide the energy source for a variety of activities important in a bird's life, in addition to the activity of breathing. Some of these will now be considered briefly.

1. Sound Production

For an animal to vocalize, a gas stream, generated by the contraction of the respiratory muscles, moving past a vocal organ is required. Most vocalization in birds occurs during expiration and the action of the expiratory muscles is precisely controlled during that act. Electromyographic recordings from the abdominal muscles during vocalization indicate rapid onset of activity, which varies with the type of sound produced.[186-192] These muscles twitch and relax up to 40 to 50 times per second during each sound pulse in the trill of awake Chicks and Canaries indicating that the active muscle fibers must have the capability of very rapid contraction and relaxation (contraction time would have to be between 10 and 20 msec).[191,193] In addition, during the crow of the Chicken, air-sac pressures as high as 60 cmH_2O have been recorded[189,194,195] and during vocalization in the Ring Dove (*Streptopelia risoria*) and Starling (*Sturnus vulgaris*), these pressures reach at least 35 cmH_2O.[192,196] During crowing in the Chicken, most of the gas appears to be removed from the air sacs by the strong expiratory effort.[195,197,198]

In these acts, it is supposed that large motor units are recruited, which can generate large tensions, in addition to the smaller motor units used during breathing. These large motor units may be used only during nonrespiratory actions and there is evidence that they are not recruited at other times.[187,191] As seen in Section II.B.1, the histochemical characteristics of the various fibers of the abdominal muscles are consistent with a wide variety of functions for these muscles.

2. Coughing and Defecation

Except for vocalization, very few studies have considered the action of the avian respiratory muscles in nonbreathing events. However, it is known that air-sac pressures also become very high (up to 30 cmH_2O) in Chickens and Geese during coughing and defecation.[195] Furthermore, the rapid rise in pressure suggests a fast contraction of the expiratory muscles in which large motor units are recruited, much like that during crowing in Chickens or honking in Geese. Thus, the behavior of these muscles appears to be similar in all those nonrespiratory actions that require high pressures in the air sacs for their success.

ACKNOWLEDGMENTS

Special appreciation is extended to Drs. Julian Baumel, James Breazile, Robert Klemm, and Robert Raikow for their helpful comments on the manuscript. This chapter was written while the author was on sabbatical leave at the Institut für Physiologie, Ruhr-Universität, Bochum, Federal Republic of Germany. Support for this effort was provided by Senior International Fellowship 1 FOG TW 00876-01 from the Department of Health and Human Services, by Grant PCM-8320260 from the National Science Foundation, and by the Alexander von Humboldt-Stiftung, Contribution no. 85-397-B, Department of Anatomy and Physiology, College of Veterinary Medicine, Kansas Agricultural Experiment Station, Manhattan, Kansas.

REFERENCES

1. **Vanden Barge, J. C.,** Myologia, in *Nomina Anatomica Avium,* Baumel, J. J., Ed., Academic Press, New York, 1979, 175.
2. **Gurlt, E. F.,** *Anatomie der Hausvögel,* August Hirschwald, Berlin, 1849.
3. **Magnus, H.,** Physiologisch-anatomische Studien über die Brust- und Bauchmuskeln der Vögel, *Arch. Anat. Physiol.,* 2, 207, 1869.

4. **Gadow, H. and Selenka, E.,** *Bronn's Klassen und Ordnungen des Thier-Reichs, Vögel, Section 4,* Vol. 6 (Part 1), C. F. Winter'sche Verlagshandlung, Leipzig, 1891.
5. **Marshall, M. E.,** A study of the anatomy of *Phalaenoptilus,* Ridgway, *Proc. Am. Phil. Soc.,* 44, 213, 1905.
6. **Kaupp, B. F.,** *Anatomy of the Domestic Fowl,* W. B. Saunders, Philadelphia, 1918.
7. **Chamberlain, F. W.,** *Atlas of Avian Anatomy,* Michigan State College Agricultural Experiment Station, Memoir Bulletin 5, East Lansing, 1943.
8. **Harvey, E. B., Kaiser, H. E., and Rosenberg, L. E.,** An Atlas of the Domestic Turkey (*Meleagris gallopavo*): Myology and Osteology, Publ. WASH 1123 TID US 48, U.S. Atomic Energy Commission, Washington, D.C., 1968.
9. **Fisher, H. I. and Goodman, D. C.,** The Myology of the Whooping Crane, *Grus Americana, Illinois Biol. Monogr.,* 24(2), 1955.
10. **Berger, A. J.,** The musculature, in *Biology and Comparative Physiology of Birds,* Vol. 1, Marshall, A. J., Ed., Academic Press, New York, 1960, chap. 8.
11. **Bradley, O. C. and Grahame, T.,** *The Structure of the Fowl,* 4th ed., Oliver and Boyd, Edinburgh, 1960.
12. **Evans, H. E.,** *Guide to the Study and Dissection of the Chicken,* New York State Veterinary College, Cornell University, Ithaca, N.Y., 1961.
13. **McLeod, W. M., Trotter, D. M., and Lumb, J. W.,** *Avian Anatomy,* Burgess, Minneapolis, 1964, 36.
14. **Hudson, G. E. and Lanzillotti, P. J.,** Muscles of the pectoral limb in galliform birds, *Am. Midl. Nat.,* 71, 1, 1964.
15. **George, J. C. and Berger, A. J.,** *Avian Myology,* Academic Press, New York, 1966.
16. **Nickel, R., Schummer, A., Seiferle, E., Siller, W. G., and Wight, P. A. L.,** *Anatomy of the Domestic Birds,* Verlag Paul Parey, Berlin, 1977, 26.
17. **deWet, P. D.,** Anatomical and Physiological Investigations of the Avian Respiratory Muscles, Ph.D. thesis, University of Minnesota, Minneapolis, 1966.
18. **deWet, P. D., Fedde, M. R., and Kitchell, R. L.,** Innervation of the respiratory muscles of *Gallus domesticus, J. Morphol.,* 123, 17, 1967.
19. **Vanden Berge, J. C.,** Aves myology, in *Sisson and Grossman's The Anatomy of the Domestic Animals,* Vol. 2, 5th ed., Getty, R., Ed., W. B. Saunders, Philadelphia, 1975, 1802.
20. **Perrault,** Memoires pour servir a l'histoire naturelle des animaux, *Mem. Acad. R. Sci.,* 3(2), 110, 1666.
21. **Hunter, J.,** An account of certain receptacles of air, in birds, which communicate with the lungs, and are lodged both among the fleshly parts and in the hollow bones of those animals, *Phil. Trans.,* 64 (I), 205, 1774.
22. **Philomathitsky, A.,** De Avium Respiration, Dissertatio Inauguralis Anatomico-Physiologica, de Universitate Caesarea Litterari, Dorpati, 1833.
23. **Owen, R.,** On the anatomy of the southern apteryx (*Apteryx australis,* Shaw), *Trans. Zool. Soc. London,* 2 (4), 257, 1842.
24. **Guillot, N.,** Mémoire sur l'appareil de la respiration dans les oiseaux, *Ann. Sci. Nat. Sér. 3 Zoologie,* 5, 25, 1846.
25. **Sappey, P. C.,** *Recherches sur L'Appareil Respiratoire des Oiseaux,* Baillière, Paris, 1847.
26. **Tigri, A.,** Del muscolo diaframma negli uccelli, *Atti Accad. Gioenia,* 5 (Ser. 3), 177, 1871.
27. **Huxley, T. H.,** On the respiratory organs of *Apteryx, Proc. Zool. Soc. London,* 560, 1882.
28. **Weldon, W. F. R.,** On some points in the anatomy of *Phoenicopterus* and its allies, *Trans. Zool. Soc. London,* Dec. 18., 638, 1883.
29. **Soum, J. M.,** Recherches physiologiques sur l'appareil respiratoire des oiseaux, *Ann. Univ. Lyon,* 28, 1, 1896.
30. **Cavalié, M.,** Innervation du diaphragme par les nerfs intercostaux chez les mammifères et chez les oiseaux, *J. Anat. Physiol.,* 34, 642, 1898.
31. **Bertelli, D.,** Sullo sviluppo del diaframma, dei sacchi aeriferi e della cavità pleuro-peritoneale nel Gallo domestico, *Monit. Zool. Ital.,* 15(9), 285, 1904.
32. **Bertelli, D.,** Ricerche de embriologia e di anatomia comparata sul diaframma e sull' apparecchio respiratorio dei vertebrati, *Arch. Ital. Anat. Embriol.,* 4, 776, 1905.
33. **Müller, B.,** The air-sacs of the pigeon, *Smithson. Misc. Collect.,* 50, 365, 1907-08.
34. **Juillet, A.,** Face ventrale du poumon des oiseaux et diaphragme, *C. R. Soc. Biol.,* 71, 230, 1911.
35. **Juillet, A.,** Recherches anatomiques, embryologiques, histologiques et comparatives sur le poumon des oiseaux, *Arch. Zool. Exp. Gen. Notes Rev.,* 5 Ser., (9), 207, 1912.
36. **Swindle, P. F.,** Mechanical factors contributing to the exchange of fluids in the body. IV. In the lungs and the ascending branches of the descending thoracic aorta of the bird, *Am. J. Physiol.,* 93, 616, 1930.
37. **Goodrich, E. S.,** *Studies on the Structure and Development of Vertebrates,* Macmillan, London, 1930, chap. 12.
38. **Fedde, M. R., Burger, R. E., and Kitchell, R. L.,** Anatomic and electromyographic studies of the costopulmonary muscles in the cock, *Poult. Sci.,* 43, 1177, 1964.

39. **Duncker, H.-R.,** Coelomic cavities, in *Form and Function in Birds,* Vol. 1, King, A. S. and McLelland, J., Eds., Academic Press, New York, 1979, 39.

40. **Duncker, H.-R.,** Functional anatomy of the respiratory system, in *Acta XVII Congressus Internationalis Ornithologici,* Vol. 1, Nöhring, R., Ed., Verlag der Deutschen Ornithologen-Gesellschaft, Berlin, 1980, 350.

41. **Zimmer, K.,** Beiträge zur Mechanik der Atmung bei den Vögeln in Stand und Flug auf Grund anatomisch-physiologischer und experimenteller Studien, *Zoologica,* 33, 5 Heft 88, 1, 1935.

42. **Chinoy, N. J. and George, J. C.,** Cellular organization and certain histophysiological features of the avian abdominal musculature, *Pavo,* 2, 12, 1964.

43. **Rawles, M. E. and Straus, W. L., Jr.,** An experimental analysis of the development of the trunk musculature and ribs in the chick, *Anat. Rec.,* 100, 755, 1948.

44. **Liebe, W.,** Das männliche Begattungsorgan der Hausente, *Jena. Z. Naturwiss.,* 51, 627, 1914.

45. **Hess, A.,** Structural differences of fast and slow extrafusal muscle fibres and their nerve endings in chickens, *J. Physiol. (London),* 157, 221, 1961.

46. **Ginsborg, B. L. and Mackay, B.,** A histochemical demonstration of two types of motor innervation in avian skeletal muscle, *Bibl. Anat.,* 2, 174, 1961.

47. **Silver, A.,** A histochemical investigation of cholinesterases at neuromuscular junctions in mammalian and avian muscle, *J. Physiol. (London),* 169, 386, 1963.

48. **Page, S. and Slater, C. R.,** Observations on fine structure and rate of contraction of some muscles from the chicken, *J. Physiol. (London),* 179, 58P, 1965.

49. **Nene, R. V. and Chinoy, N. J.,** Histochemical observations on the avian Mm. latissimus dorsi, anterior and posterior, *Pavo,* 3, 29, 1965.

50. **Mayr, R.,** Zur elektronenmikroskopischen Unterscheidbarkeit eines einfach und eines multipel innervierten Hühnermuskels, *Naturwissenschaften,* 54, 22, 1967.

51. **Hess, A.,** The structure of vertebrate slow and twitch muscle fibers, *Invest. Ophthalmol.,* 6, 217, 1967.

52. **Zelená, J., Vyklický, L., and Jirmanová, I.,** Motor end-plates in fast and slow muscles of the chick after cross-union of their nerves, *Nature,* 214, 1010, 1967.

53. **Gutmann, E., Hanzlíková, V., and Holečková, E.,** Development of fast and slow muscles of the chicken in vivo and their latent period in tissue culture, *Exp. Cell Res.,* 56, 33, 1969.

54. **Asmussen, G., Kiessling, A., and Wohlrab, F.,** Histochemisch differenzierbare Sorten von Muskelfasern im M. latissimus dorsi des Huhnes, *Experientia,* 25, 959, 1969.

55. **Page, S. G.,** Structure and some contractile properties of fast and slow muscles of the chicken, *J. Physiol. (London),* 205, 131, 1969.

56. **Jirmanová, I. and Zelená, J.,** Effect of denervation and tenotomy on slow and fast muscles of the chicken, *Z. Zellforsch.,* 106, 333, 1970.

57. **Shear, C. R. and Goldspink, G.,** Structural and physiological changes associated with the growth of avian fast and slow muscle, *J. Morphol.,* 135, 351, 1971.

58. **Ashmore, C. R. and Doerr, L.,** Postnatal development of fiber types in normal and dystrophic skeletal muscle of the chick, *Exp. Neurol.,* 30, 431, 1971.

59. **Hikida, R. S. and Bock, W. J.,** Innervation of the avian tonus latissimus dorsi anterior muscle, *Am. J. Anat.,* 130, 269, 1971.

60. **Hikida, R. S. and Bock, W. J.,** Effect of denervation on pigeon slow skeletal muscle, *Z. Zellforsch.,* 128, 1, 1972.

61. **Asiedu, S. and Shafiq, S. A.,** Actomyosin ATPase activity of the anterior latissimus dorsi muscle of the chicken, *Exp. Neurol.,* 35, 211, 1972.

62. **Wilson, B. W., Linkhart, S. G., and Nieberg, P. A.,** Acetylcholinesterase in singly and multiply innervated muscles of normal and dystrophic chickens, *J. Exp. Zool.,* 186, 187, 1973.

63. **Zelená, J. and Jirmanová, I.,** Ultrastructure of chicken slow muscle after nerve cross union, *Exp. Neurol.,* 38, 272, 1973.

64. **Koenig, J. and Fardeau, M.,** Étude histochemique des muscles grands dorsaux antérieur et postérieur du poulet et des modifications observées après dénervation et réinnervation homologue ou croisée, *Arch. Anat. Microsc.,* 62, 249, 1973.

65. **Jirmanová, I. and Zelená, J.,** Ultrastructural transformation of fast chicken muscle fibres induced by nerve cross-union, *Z. Zellforsch.,* 146, 103, 1973.

66. **Gordon, T., Perry, R., Tuffery, A. R., and Vrbová, G.,** Possible mechanisms determining synapse formation in developing skeletal muscles of the chick, *Cell Tissue Res.,* 155, 13, 1974.

67. **Ovalle, W. K.,** Extrafusal and intrafusal fiber types in a vertebrate slow (tonic) muscle, *Anat. Rec.,* 181, 441, 1975.

68. **Khan, M. A.,** Histochemical characteristics of vertebrate striated muscle: a review, *Prog. Histochem. Cytochem.,* 8, 1, 1976.

69. **Ovalle, W. K.,** Fine structure of the avian muscle spindle capsule, *Cell Tissue Res.,* 166, 285, 1976.

70. **Ashmore, C. R. and Doerr, L.,** Transplantation of the anterior latissimus dorsi muscle in normal and dystrophic chickens, *Exp. Neurol.,* 50, 312, 1976.
71. **Burden, S.,** Development of the neuromuscular junction in the chick embryo: the number, distribution, and stability of acetylcholine receptors, *Dev. Biol.,* 57, 317, 1977.
72. **Atsumi, S.,** Development of neuromuscular junctions of fast and slow muscles in the chick embryo: a light and electron microscopic study, *J. Neurocytol.,* 6, 691, 1977.
73. **Gordon, T., Perry, R., Srihari, T., and Vrbová, G.,** Differentiation of slow and fast muscles in chickens, *Cell Tissue Res.,* 180, 211, 1977.
74. **Ovalle, W. K., Jr.,** Histochemical dichotomy of extrafusal and intrafusal fibers in an avian slow muscle, *Am. J. Anat.,* 152, 587, 1978.
75. **Ashmore, C. R., Kikuchi, T., and Doerr, L.,** Some observations on the innervation patterns of different fiber types of chick muscle, *Exp. Neurol.,* 58, 272, 1978.
76. **Toutant, J. P., Toutant, M. N., Renaud, D., and Le Douarin, G. H.,** Enzymatic differentiation of muscle fibre types in embryonic *latissimus dorsii* of the chick: effects of spinal cord stimulation, *Cell Differ.,* 8, 375, 1979.
77. **Toutant, J. P., Toutant, M. N., Renaud, D., and Le Douarin, G. H.,** Histochemical differentiation of extrafusal muscle fibres of the *anterior latissimus dorsi* in the chick, *Cell Differ.,* 9, 305, 1980.
78. **Toutant, M., Bourgeois, J.-P., Toutant, J.-P., Renaud, D., Le Douarin, G., and Changeux, J.-P.,** Chronic stimulation of the spinal cord in developing chick embryo causes the differentiation of multiple clusters of acetylcholine receptor in the posterior latissimus dorsi muscle, *Dev. Biol.,* 76, 384, 1980.
79. **Toutant, M., Toutant, J. P., Renaud, D., and Le Douarin, G.,** Effects of spinal cord stimulation on the differentiation of posterior latissimus dorsi nerve in the chick embryo, *Exp. Neurol.,* 72, 267, 1981.
80. **Gray, S. D., McDonagh, P. F., and Gore, R. W.,** Comparison of functional and total capillary densities in fast and slow muscles of the chicken., *Pflügers Arch.,* 397, 209, 1983.
81. **Peter, J. B., Barnard, R. J., Edgerton, V. R., Gillespie, C. A., and Stempel, K. E.,** Metabolic profiles of three fiber types of skeletal muscle in guinea pigs and rabbits, *Biochemistry,* 11, 2627, 1972.
82. **Burke, R. E. and Tsairis, P.,** The correlation of physiological properties with histochemical characteristics in single muscle units, *Ann. N. Y. Acad. Sci.,* 228, 145, 1974.
83. **Burke, R. E.,** Motor units: anatomy, physiology, and functional organization, in *Handbook of Physiology, The Nervous System,* Section 1, Vol. 2, *Motor Control,* Part 1, Brooks, V. B., Ed., American Physiological Society, Bethesda, Md., 1981, chap. 10.
84. **Saltin, B. and Gollnick, P. D.,** Skeletal muscle adaptability: significance for metabolism and performance, in *Handbook of Physiology. Skeletal Muscle,* Section 10, Peachey, L. D., Ed., American Physiological Soc., Bethesda, Md., 1983, chap. 19.
85. **Khan, M. A.,** Histochemical sub-types of three fibre-types of avian skeletal muscle, *Histochemistry,* 50, 9, 1976.
86. **Farrell, P. R. and Fedde, M. R.,** Uniformity of structural characteristics throughout the length of skeletal muscle fibers, *Anat. Rec.,* 164, 219, 1969.
87. **Fedde, M. R. and Cardinet, G. H., III,** Histochemical studies of respiratory muscles of chicken, *Am. J. Vet. Res.,* 38, 585, 1977.
88. **Guth, L.,** ''Trophic'' influences of nerve on muscle, *Physiol. Rev.,* 48, 645, 1968.
89. **Matthews, P. B. C.,** Evolving views on the internal operation and functional role of the muscle spindle, *J. Physiol. (London),* 320, 1, 1981.
90. **Huber, G. C. and DeWitt, L. M. A.,** A contribution on the motor nerve-endings and on the nerve-endings in the muscle-spindles, *J. Comp. Neurol.,* 7, 169, 1898.
91. **Cipollone, L. T.,** Ricerche sull'anatomia normale e patologica delle terminazioni nervose nei muscoli striati, *Ann. Med. Nav. Colon.,* Suppl. 3, 223, 1897.
92. **Tello, J. F.,** Génesis de las terminaciones nerviosas motrices y sensitivas. I. En el sistema locomotor de los vertebrados superiores. Histogenesis muscular, *Trab. Lab. Invest. Biol. Univ. Madrid,* 15, 101, 1917.
93. **Shehata, S. H.,** The Innervation of Avian Muscles, Ph.D. thesis, Royal Free Hospital School of Medicine, London, 1961.
94. **Sağlam, M.,** Morphologische und quantitative Untersuchungen über die Muskelspindeln in der Nacken-muskulatur (M. biventer cervicis, M. rectus capitis dorsalis und M. rectus capitis lateralis) des Bunt- und Blutspechtes, *Acta Anat.,* 69, 87, 1968.
95. **Maier, A., De Santis, M., and Eldred, E.,** Absence of muscle spindles in avian extraocular muscles, *Exp. Eye Res.,* 12, 251, 1971.
96. **Veggetti, A. and Palmieri, G.,** Distribution, frequency and morphology of muscle spindle of the masticatory muscles in some domestic birds, *Riv. Biol.,* 64, 215, 1971.
97. **Maier, A. and Eldred, E.,** Comparisons in the structure of avian muscle spindles, *J. Comp. Neurol.,* 143, 25, 1971.
98. **Maier, A., DeSantis, M., and Eldred, E.,** The occurrence of muscle spindles in extraocular muscles of various vertebrates, *J. Morphol.,* 143, 397, 1974.

99. **Adal, M. N. and Cheng Chew, S.-B.,** Spindles in some wing muscles of the domestic duck, *J. Anat.,* 119, 202, 1975.
100. **Maier, A., Eldred, E., and Burton, R. R.,** Effects of long-term increased gravitational load on intrafusal fibers on the avian muscle spindle, *Brain Res.,* 112, 180, 1976.
101. **Lippock, R.,** Anatomie, Anzahl und Verteilung von Muskelspindeln in der Stellmuskulatur des Unterarms der Amsel (*Turdus merula* L.), Diplomarbeit, Institut für Allgemeine Zoologie, Freie Universität Berlin, Berlin, 1977.
102. **Bilo, D., Jahner, A., and Nachtigall, W.,** Structure and innervation of wing muscle spindles in the domestic pigeon (*Columba livia* var. *domestica*); a light microscopical study, *Zool. Jahrb. Anat.,* 103, 41, 1980.
103. **Maier, A.,** Characteristics of pigeon gastrocnemius and its muscle spindle supply, *Exp. Neurol.,* 74, 892, 1981.
104. **Maier, A.,** Differences in muscle spindle structure between pigeon muscles used in aerial and terrestrial locomotion, *Am. J. Anat.,* 168, 27, 1983.
105. **De Anda, G. and Rebollo, M. A.,** The neuromuscular spindles in the adult chicken. I. Morphology, *Acta Anat.,* 67, 437, 1967.
106. **Germino, N. I. and D'Albora, H.,** Succinic-dehydrogenase activity in the neuromuscular spindles of the chick, *Experientia,* 21, 45, 1965.
107. **Rebollo, M. A. and De Anda, G.,** The neuromuscular spindles in the adult chicken. II. Histochemistry, *Acta Anat.,* 67, 595, 1967.
108. **Maier, A.,** Variations in intrafusal fiber size within histochemically identified types of intrafusal fibers in the pigeon, *Am. J. Anat.,* 150, 375, 1977.
109. **Toutant, M., Bourgeois, J. P., Rouaud, T., and Toutant, J. P.,** Morphological and histochemical differentiation of intrafusal fibres in the *posterior latissimus dorsi* muscle of the developing chick, *Anat. Embryol.,* 162, 325, 1981.
110. **Toutant, M.,** Quantitative and histochemical aspects of the differentiation of muscle spindles in the anterior latissimus dorsi of the developing chick, *Anat. Embryol.,* 163, 475, 1982.
111. **James, N. T. and Meek, G. A.,** The ultrastructure of the avian muscle spindle, *J. Anat.,* 111, 489, 1972.
112. **James, N. T. and Meek, G. A.,** An electron microscopical study of avian muscle spindles, *J. Ultrastruct. Res.,* 43, 193, 1973.
113. **Adal, M. N.,** The fine structure of the intrafusal muscle fibres of muscle spindles in the domestic fowl, *J. Anat.,* 115, 407, 1973.
114. **Adal, M. N.,** Leptofibrils in intrafusal muscle fibres of muscle spindles in the domestic fowl, *Cell Tissue Res.,* 184, 281, 1977.
115. **Chin, N. K.,** Innervation of chicken muscle spindles, *J. Anat.,* 119, 203, 1975.
116. **Manzij, S. F. and Sytsch, W. F.,** Zur Morphologie sensorischer intramuskulärer Innervation der Flügelmuskeln bei den Vögeln, *Zool. Jahrb. Anat.,* 100, 3, 1978.
117. **Adal, M. N. and Chew Cheng, S. B.,** The sensory ending of duck muscle spindles, *J. Anat.,* 131, 657, 1980.
118. **Maier, A.,** The blood supply of muscle spindles in some mammals and the pigeon, *J. Morphol.,* 161, 323, 1979.
119. **deWet, P. D., Farrell, P. R., and Fedde, M. R.,** Number and morphology of muscle spindles in the *transversus abdominis* muscle of the chicken, *Poult. Sci.,* 50, 1349, 1971.
120. **Sears, T. A.,** Efferent discharges of alpha fusimotor fibres of intercostal nerves of the cat, *J. Physiol. (London),* 174, 295, 1964.
121. **Bridgman, C. F., Shumpert, E. E., and Eldred, E.,** Insertions of intrafusal fibers in muscle spindles of the cat and other mammals, *Anat. Rec.,* 164, 391, 1969.
122. **Gray, S. D. and Renkin, E. M.,** Microvascular supply in relation to fiber metabolic type in mixed skeletal muscles in rabbits, *Microvasc. Res.,* 16, 406, 1978.
123. **Krogh, A.,** *The Anatomy and Physiology of Capillaries,* Yale University Press, New Haven, Conn., 1922.
124. **Hoppeler, H., Mathieu, O., Weibel, E. R., Krauer, R., Lindstedt, S. L., and Taylor, C. R.,** Design of the mammalian respiratory system. VIII. Capillaries in skeletal muscles, *Respir. Physiol.,* 44, 129, 1981.
125. **Ginsborg, B. L.,** Some properties of avian skeletal muscle fibres with multiple neuromuscular junctions, *J. Physiol. (London),* 154, 581, 1960.
126. **Ginsborg, B. L.,** Spontaneous activity in muscle fibres of the chick, *J. Physiol. (London),* 150, 707, 1960.
127. **Hník, P., Jirmanová, I., Vyklický, L., and Zelená, J.,** Fast and slow muscles of the chick after nerve cross-union, *J. Physiol. London,* 193, 309, 1967.
128. **Fedde, M. R.,** Electrical properties and acetylcholine sensitivity of singly and multiply innervated avian muscle fibers, *J. Gen. Physiol.,* 53, 624, 1969.
129. **Hudlická, O.,** Resting and postcontraction blood flow in slow and fast muscles of the chick during development, *Microvasc. Res.,* 1, 390, 1969.

130. **Goldspink, G., Larson, R. E., and Davies, R. E.,** Thermodynamic efficiency and physiological characteristics of the chick anterior latissimus dorsi muscle, *Z. Vgl. Physiol.,* 66, 379, 1970.

131. **Gutmann, E., Hájek, I., and Vítek, V.,** Compensatory hypertrophy of the latissimus dorsi posterior muscle induced by elimination of the latissimus dorsi anterior muscle of the chicken, *Physiol. Bohemoslov.,* 19, 483, 1970.

132. **Canfield, S. P.,** The mechanical properties and heat production of chicken latissimus dorsi muscles during tetanic contractions, *J. Physiol. (London),* 219, 281, 1971.

133. **Vyskočil, F., Vyklický, L., and Huston, R.,** Quantum content at the neuromuscular junction of fast muscle after cross-union with the nerve of slow muscle in the chick, *Brain Res.,* 26, 443, 1971.

134. **Fedde, M. R.,** Contractile characteristics of fast and slow skeletal muscles, *Physiol. Teacher,* 2, 2, 1973.

135. **Sola, O. M., Christensen, D. L., and Martin, A. W.,** Hypertrophy and hyperplasia of adult chicken anterior latissimus dorsi muscles following stretch with and without denervation, *Exp. Neurol.,* 41, 76, 1973.

136. **Bennett, M. R., Pettigrew, A. G., and Taylor, R. S.,** The formation of synapses in reinnervated and cross-reinnervated adult avian muscle, *J. Physiol. London,* 230, 331, 1973.

137. **Melichna, J., Gutmann, E., and Syrový, I.,** Developmental changes in contraction properties, adenosine-triphosphatase activity and muscle fibre pattern of fast and slow chicken muscle, *Physiol. Bohemoslov.,* 23, 511, 1974.

138. **Purves, R. D. and Vrbová, G.,** Some characteristics of myotubes cultured from slow and fast chick muscles, *J. Cell. Physiol.,* 84, 97, 1974.

139. **Vyskočil, F. and Vklický, L.,** Acetylcholine sensitivity of the chick fast muscle after cross-union with the slow muscle nerve, *Brain Res.,* 72, 158, 1974.

140. **Gordon, T. and Vrbová, G.,** The influence of innervation on the differentiation of contractile speeds of developing chick muscles, *Pflügers Arch.,* 360, 199, 1975.

141. **Klabunde, R. E. and Johnson, P. C.,** Reactive hyperemia in capillaries of red and white skeletal muscle, *Am. J. Physiol.,* 232, H411, 1977.

142. **McDonagh, P. F. and Gore, R. W.,** Comparison of hydraulic conductivities in single capillaries of red versus white skeletal muscle, *Microvasc. Res.,* 15, 269, 1978.

143. **Renaud, D., LeDouarin, G. H., and Khaskiye, A.,** Spinal cord stimulation in chick embryo: effects on development of the posterior latissimus dorsi muscle and neuromuscular junctions, *Exp. Neurol.,* 60, 189, 1978.

144. **McDonagh, P. F., Gore, R. W., Gray, S. D., and Ferrer, P.,** Perfused capillary surface area in tonic and phasic skeletal muscles, *Microvasc. Res.,* 20, 119, 1980.

145. **McDonagh, P. F., Gore, R. W., and Gray, S. D.,** Perfused capillary surface area in postural and locomotor skeletal muscle, *Microvasc. Res.,* 24, 142, 1982.

146. **Chang, C. and Feng, T.-P.,** Comparative study on the protein and nucleic acid changes of the anterior and posterior latissimus dorsi of the chick following denervation, *Acta Physiol. Sin. Abstr.,* 25, 312, 1962.

147. **Feng, T.-P., Jung, H.-W., and Wu, W.-Y.,** The contrasting trophic changes of the anterior and posterior latissimus dorsi of the chick following denervation, *Acta Physiol. Sin. Abstr.,* 25, 304, 1962.

148. **Syrový, I. and Gutmann, E.,** Metabolic differentiation of the anterior and posterior latissimus dorsi of the chick during development, *Nature,* 213, 937, 1967.

149. **Gutmann, E. and Syrový, I.,** Metabolic differentiation of the anterior and posterior latissimus dorsi of the chicken during development, *Physiol. Bohemoslov.,* 16, 232, 1967.

150. **Bass, A., Brdiczka, D., Eyer, P., Hofer, S., and Pette, D.,** Metabolic differentiation of distinct muscle types at the level of enzymatic organization, *Eur. J. Biochem.,* 10, 198, 1969.

151. **Bass, A., Lusch, G., and Pette, D.,** Postnatal differentiation of the enzyme activity pattern of energy-supplying metabolism in slow (red) and fast (white) muscles of chick, *Eur. J. Biochem.,* 13, 289, 1970.

152. **Reasons, R. H. and Hikida, R. S.,** Biochemistry of adenosine triphosphatase activity of avian fast and slow muscle, *Exp. Neurol.,* 38, 27, 1973.

153. **Masaki, T.,** Immunochemical comparison of myosins from chicken cardiac, fast white, slow red, and smooth muscle, *J. Biochem.,* 76, 441, 1974.

154. **Arndt, I. and Pepe, F. A.,** Antigenic specificity of red and white muscle myosin, *J. Histochem. Cytochem.,* 23, 159, 1975.

155. **Hudlická, O.,** Uptake of substrates in slow and fast muscles *in situ, Microvasc. Res.,* 10, 17, 1975.

156. **Hoh, J. F. Y., McGrath, P. A., and White, R. I.,** Electrophoretic analysis of multiple forms of myosin in fast-twitch and slow-twitch muscles of the chick, *Biochem. J.,* 157, 87, 1976.

157. **Betz, H., Bourgeois, J.-P., and Changeux, J.-P.,** Evidence for degradation of the acetylcholine (nicotinic) receptor in skeletal muscle during the development of the chick embryo, *FEBS Lett.,* 77, 219, 1977.

158. **O'Brien, R. A. D. and Vrbová, G.,** Acetylcholine synthesis in nerve endings to slow and fast muscles of developing chicks: effects of muscle activity, *Neuroscience,* 3, 1227, 1978.

159. **Klabunde, R. E. and Mayer, S. E.,** Effects of ischemia on tissue metabolites in red (slow) and white (fast) skeletal muscle of the chicken, *Circ. Res.,* 45, 366, 1979.

160. **Betz, H., Bourgeois, J.-P., and Changeux, J.-P.,** Evolution of cholinergic proteins in developing slow and fast skeletal muscles in chick embryo, *J. Physiol. (London),* 302, 197, 1980.

161. **Faraci, F. M.,** Control of the Circulation in High and Low Altitude Adapted Birds, Ph.D. thesis, Kansas State University, Manhattan, 1984.

162. **Sibson, F.,** On the mechanism of respiration, *Philos. Trans. R. Soc. London,* p. 501, 1846.

163. **Campana, A.,** *Physiologie de la respiration chez les Oiseaux anatomie de l'appareil pneumonique-pulmonaire, des faux-diaphragmes, des sereuses et de l'intestin chez le poulet,* Masson, Paris, 1875.

164. **Headley, F. W.,** The respiration of birds, *Natural Sci.,* 3, 28, 1893.

165. **Baer, M.,** Beiträge zur Kenntnis der Anatomie und Physiologie der Athemwerkzeuge bei den Vögeln, *Z. Wiss. Zool. Abt. A,* 61, 420, 1896.

166. **Babák, E.,** Die Mechanik und Innervation der Atmung, in *Handbuch der vergleichenden Physiologie,* Vol. 1 (Part 2), Winterstein, H., Ed., Fischer, Jena, 1921, 880.

167. **Burkart, F. and Bucher, K.,** Elektromyographische Untersuchungen an der Atmungsmuskulatur der Taube, *Helv. Physiol. Acta,* 19, 263, 1961.

168. **Kadono, H. and Okada, T.,** Electromyographic studies on the respiratory muscles of the domestic fowl, *Jpn. J. Vet. Sci.,* 24, 215, 1962.

169. **Kadono, H., Okada, T., and Ono, K.,** Electromyographic studies on the respiratory muscles of the chicken, *Poult. Sci.,* 42, 121, 1963.

170. **Fedde, M. R., Burger, R. E., and Kitchell, R. L.,** Electromyographic studies on certain respiratory muscles of the chicken, *Poult. Sci.,* 42, 1269, 1963.

171. **Fedde, M. R., Burger, R. E., and Kitchell, R. L.,** Electromyographic studies of the effects of bodily position and anesthesia on the activity of the respiratory muscles of the domestic cock, *Poult. Sci.,* 43, 839, 1964.

172. **Fedde, M. R., Burger, R. E., and Kitchell, R. L.,** Electromyographic studies of the effects of bilateral, cervical vagotomy on the action of the respiratory muscles of the domestic cock, *Poult. Sci.,* 43, 1119, 1964.

173. **Jones, J. H., Effmann, E. L., and Schmidt-Nielsen, K.,** Lung volume changes during respiration in ducks, *Respir. Physiol.,* 59, 15, 1985.

174. **King, A. S. and Payne, D. C.,** Normal breathing and the effects of posture in *Gallus domesticus, J., Physiol. (London),* 174, 340, 1964.

175. **Kuhlmann, W. D. and Fedde, M. R.,** unpublished data, 1985.

176. **Fedde, M. R.,** Drugs used for avian anesthesia: a review, *Poult. Sci.,* 57, 1376, 1978.

177. **Fedde, M. R., Burger, R. E., and Kitchell, R. L.,** The effect of anesthesia and age on respiration following bilateral, cervical vagotomy in the fowl, *Poultry Sci.,* 42, 1212, 1963.

178. **King, A. S.,** Afferent pathways in the vagus and their influence on avian breathing: a review, in *Physiology of the Domestic Fowl,* Horton-Smith, C. and Amoroso, E. C., Eds., Oliver and Boyd, London, 1966, 302.

179. **Hambolu, J. O., Schumacher, K. G., and Fedde, M. R.,** Breathing pattern in anesthetized chickens: CO_2 inhalation and vagotomy, *Comp. Biochem. Physiol.,* 81A, 185, 1985.

180. **Henneman, E. and Mendell, L. M.,** Functional organization of motoneuron pool and its inputs, in *Handbook of Physiology. The Nervous System,* Section 1, Vol. II, *Motor Control,* Part 1, Brookhart, J. M. and Mountcastle, V. B., Eds., American Physiological Society, Bethesda, Md., 1981, chap. 11.

181. **Loofbourrow, G. N. and Gesell, R.,** Comparative studies of the respiratory act (activity patterns), *Am. J. Physiol.,* 133, P365, 1941.

182. **Fedde, M. R., deWet, P. D., and Kitchell, R. L.,** Motor unit recruitment pattern and tonic activity in respiratory muscles of *Gallus domesticus, J. Neurophysiol.,* 32, 995, 1969.

183. **Sears, T. A.,** The activity of the small motor fibre system innervating respiratory muscles of the cat, *Aust. J. Sci.,* 25, 102, 1962.

184. **Reichow, R. W.,** Electromyography of Heterogeneous Dark and Pale Muscle, M.S. thesis, Kansas State University, Manhattan, 1967.

185. **Tschorn, R. R. and Fedde, M. R.,** Motor unit recruitment pattern in a respiratory muscle of unanesthetized chickens, *Poult. Sci.,* 50, 266, 1971.

186. **Youngren, O. M., Peek, F. W., and Phillips, R. E.,** Repetitive vocalization evoked by local electrical stimulation of avian brains. III. Evoked activity in the tracheal muscles of the chicken (*Gallus gallus*), *Brain Behav. Evol.,* 9, 393, 1974.

187. **Peek, F. W., Youngren, O. M., and Phillips, R. E.,** Repetitive vocalizations evoked by electrical stimulation of avian brains. IV. Evoked and spontaneous activity in expiratory and inspiratory nerves and muscles in the chicken (*Gallus gallus*), *Brain Behav. Evol.,* 12, 1, 1975.

188. **Lockner, F. R. and Youngren, O. M.,** Functional syringeal anatomy of the mallard. I. *In situ* electromyograms during ESB elicited calling, *Auk,* 93, 324, 1976.

189. **Gaunt, A. S., Gaunt, S. L. L., and Hector, D. H.,** Mechanics of the syrinx in *Gallus gallus.* I. A comparison of pressure events in chickens to those in oscines, *Condor,* 78, 208, 1976.

190. **Gaunt, A. S. and Gaunt, S. L. L.,** Mechanics of the syrinx in *Gallus gallus.* II. Electromyographic studies of *ad libitum* vocalizations, *J. Morphol.,* 152, 1, 1977.

191. **Phillips, R. E. and Youngren, O. M.,** Effects of denervation of the tracheo-syringeal muscles on frequency control in vocalizations in chicks, *Auk,* 98, 299, 1981.

192. **Gaunt, A. S., Gaunt, S. L. L., and Casey, R. M.,** Syringeal mechanics reassessed: evidence from *Streptopelia, Auk,* 99, 474, 1982.

193. **Calder, W. A.,** Respiration during song in the canary (*Serinus canaria*), *Comp. Biochem. Physiol.,* 32, 251, 1970.

194. **Brackenbury, J. H.,** Lung-air-sac anatomy and respiratory pressures in the bird, *J. Exp. Biol.,* 57, 543, 1972.

195. **Brackenbury, J. H.,** Respiratory mechanics of sound production in chickens and geese, *J. Exp. Biol.,* 72, 229, 1978.

196. **Gaunt, A. S., Stein, R. C., and Gaunt, S. L. L.,** Pressure and air flow during distress calls of the starling, *Sturnus vulgaris* (Aves; Passeriformes), *J. Exp. Zool.,* 183, 241, 1973.

197. **Brackenbury, J. H.,** Respiration and production of sounds by birds, *Biol. Rev.,* 55, 363, 1980.

198. **Brackenbury, J. H.,** The structural basis of voice production and its relationship to sound characteristics, in *Acoustic Communications in Birds,* Vol. 1, Kroodsma, D. E. and Miller, E. H., Eds., Academic Press, New York, 1982, 53.

199. **Baumel, J. J.,** Aves nervous system, in *Sisson and Grossman's The Anatomy of the Domestic Animals,* Vol. 2, 5th ed., Getty, R., Ed., W. B. Saunders, Philadelphia, 1975, 2019.

200. **Baumel, J. J.,** Variation in the brachial plexus of *Progne subis, Acta Anat.,* 34, 1, 1958.

201. **Buchholz, V.,** Beitrag zur makroskopischen Anatomie des Armgeflechtes und der Beckennerven beim Haushuhn (*Gallus domesticus*), *Wiss. Z. Humboldt Univ. Berlin, Math. Naturwiss Reihe,* 9, 515, 1959—60.

Chapter 2

VENTILATION OF THE LUNG-AIR SAC SYSTEM

J. H. Brackenbury

TABLE OF CONTENTS

I. INTRODUCTION

The avian lung/air sac system is much more closely related structurally to the reptilian respiratory system than it is to the lungs of mammals. It bears a strong resemblance to the multicameral lung of crocodiles, monitor lizards, and turtles,[1] although the latter never attain the complexity of structure and function seen in the bird. Birds and reptiles are also alike in possessing a costal pump but lacking a diaphragmatic pump in the mammalian sense. On the other hand, birds are unlike reptiles in being endothermic, rather than ectothermic, and in being able to sustain high aerobic metabolic rates for prolonged periods of time. In this respect they are capable of matching the top performance of exercising mammals, indicating that although the gas-exchange apparatus is markedly different in form in the two classes, there is little difference in efficiency.

The presence of air sacs connected to the lung gives the bird a large residual volume which is the basis of at least two of the most distinctive avian respiratory characteristics. First, compared to a mammal of the same body weight, a bird breathes much more slowly but also more deeply. Second, the air sacs provide a large source of air that can be used, not only in gas exchange, but also as a vehicle for heat loss by respiratory evaporation. The present chapter is concerned with the ventilation of the lung/air sac system in resting and nonresting conditions and in particular with the factors which control pulmonary airflow during thermal panting and exercise.

II. RESPIRATORY MECHANICS

A. Air Sac Pressures and Respiratory Air Flow

Owing to the absence of a muscular diaphragm homologous to that of mammals, the body cavity is not divided into two separate pressure compartments. Therefore pressure changes produced within the body cavity as a result of respiratory movements are of the same magnitude and phase in the anterior and posterior compartments into which the body cavity is divided by the posthepatic septum (Figure 1). Muscle fibers are present within the posthepatic septum, but only sparsely, and they appear to play no significant role in respiratory mechanics. Respiratory movements produce pressure fluctuations within the air sacs of the order of ± 1 cmH$_2$O, and there is no phase lag between pressure changes in the different air sacs, indicating that they expand and collapse synchronously as first described by Baer.[2] Cohn and Shannon,[3] who performed some of the first experimental measurements on avian respiration using modern transducers, concluded that there were no pressure differences between the various air sacs. However, use of highly sensitive manometers has shown the existence of a small but significant pressure gradient between the caudal (abdominal, caudal thoracic) and cranial (cervical, clavicular, cranial thoracic) groups of sacs such that the instantaneous pressures in the former are some 10% more positive than the latter during expiration and 10% more negative during inspiration. Although extremely small, this finite pressure gradient across the lung is sufficient to generate the complex pattern of intrapulmonary air flow described in Section III.

The air sac pressure and respiratory air flow waveforms are virtually identical in shape since air is driven into and out of the lung/air sac system under the bellows-like action of the air sacs. Expiration is the longer phase, and during normal breathing the expiratory air sac pressure and air flow waves show an exponential decay (Figures 2 and 3). This pattern is similar to that observed in mammalian breathing and in the latter case can be explained by the passive recoil of the lungs and rib cage. In birds, however, expiration is thought to be active under the influence of the expiratory abdominal and intercostal muscles.[4,5] This apparent inconsistency is so far unexplained. Whenever respiration is accelerated, as for example during panting or exercise, it is the expiratory period which shortens and ultimately

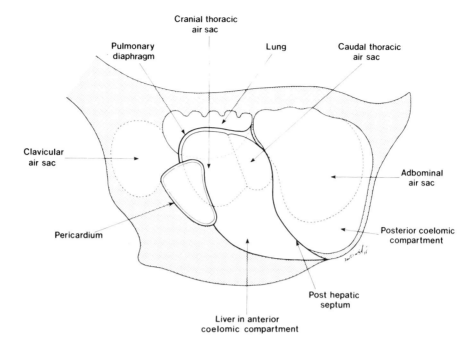

FIGURE 1.   Diagram of the relationships between the coelomic compartments and the lung/air sac system.

if respiration is sufficiently rapid, the respiratory movements become sinusoidal with inspiration and expiration being of equal duration.

The similarity between the air sac pressure and air flow waveforms (Figures 1, 2, and 3) suggests that the resistance of the lung and trachea is virtually linear. However, measurements made during normal breathing[6] and during artificial unidirectional ventilation of the lung/air sac system[7] show that airway resistance increases with air flow rate. A nonlinear relationship between pressure and air flow was found between the ventrobronchi and the dorsobronchi, between the ventrobronchi and the cranial air sacs, and between the dorsobronchi and the cranial air sacs;[7] in short, between almost any two sufficiently well-separated points within the lung. Molony et al.[7] cited the following regions as possible locations for nonlinear resistance effects: ventrobronchi, dorsobronchi, parabronchi, or the ventrobronchial and dorsobronchial orifices at their point of junction with the mesobronchus. The resistance of the dorsobronchi and of their orifices was small since the pressure measured across the lung between the dorsobronchi and ventrobronchi remained unaltered even when the dorsobronchi were opened to the atmosphere. It therefore appears that the ventrobronchial orifices may be responsible for a substantial fraction of the total pressure drop across the lung, and the difference between the intrinsic flow resistances of the dorsobronchial and ventrobronchial orifices may have important implications with regard to the determination of intrapulmonary air flow pattern.

The nonlinearity in the air sac pressure/air flow relationship is partly attributable to turbulence, but also to the geometry of the airways.[6] Whereas turbulence effects only become evident at Reynolds numbers above 2000, geometrical effects are operative at all flow rates both above and below the laminar-turbulent flow transition velocity. One of the most important geometrical flow determinants may result from the fact that air flowing along a duct with rapidly widening walls, i.e., into a diverging nozzle, encounters a smaller resistance than air flowing in the opposite direction, i.e., into a converging nozzle. It has been proposed[6] that the resistance to air flow from the caudal end of the mesobronchus into the dorsobronchi,

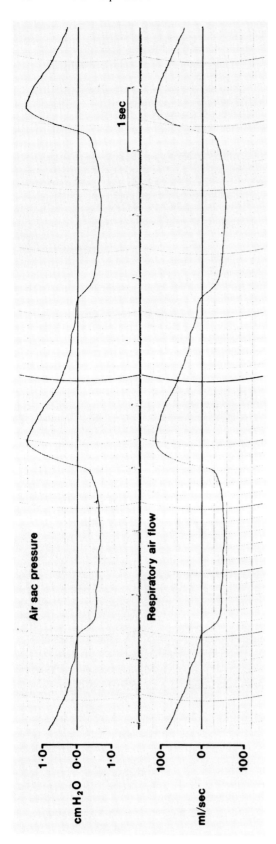

FIGURE 2.   Original recordings of air sac pressure and respiratory air flow during normal respiration in a Goose.   Pressure was recorded using a manometer and air flow using a pneumotachograph.

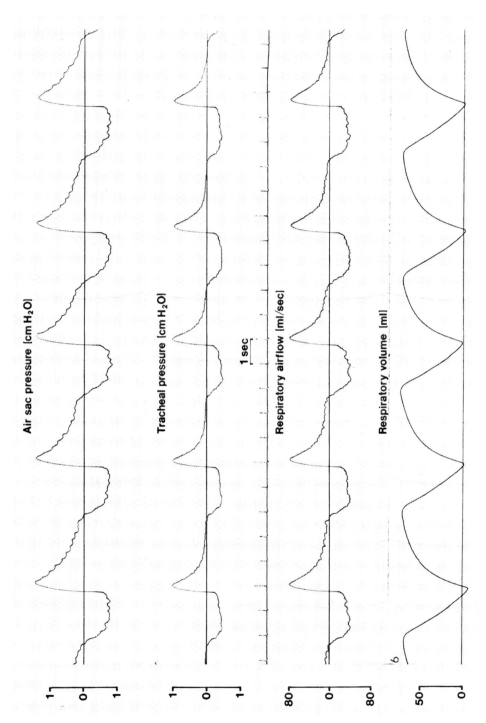

FIGURE 3.   Original recordings of air sac pressure, tracheal pressure, respiratory air flow and respiratory volume during normal respiration in a Duck.

via the dorsobronchial orifices, may be less than the resistance to air flow from the dorsobronchi into the mesobronchus, since in the former case the air must flow into an chamber whereas in the latter it would have to converge into the narrow dorsobronchial orifice (Figure 13).

During normal breathing the instantaneous tracheal pressure is rather less than that of the air sacs (Figure 3) due to a small pressure drop across the syrinx and lung. During vocalization, this drop can increase enormously as a result of the infolding of the tympaniform membranes of the syrinx. When a Domestic Cock (*Gallus gallus*) crows, the air sac pressure can rise to a maximum of approximately 60 cmH_2O, whereas tracheal pressure does not exceed approximately 15 cmH_2O (Figure 4). Thus, approximately 75% of the loss of pressure head is attributable to the passage of air through the lung and syrinx.

B. Respiratory Frequency

According to Calder[8] the lowest recorded respiratory rate in birds was 5 to 6 min^{-1} in the adult Ostrich (*Struthio camelus*), which weighs 90 to 100 kg. The Pelican (*Pelecanus erythrorhynchos*), body weight 7.5 kg, has a respiratory rate of 6.3 min^{-1}, but the lowest value must be the three breaths per min^{-1} measured in the Mute Swan (*Cygnus olor*) by Bech and Johansen.[9] The Swan also displayed an unusual respiratory pattern in which the breath was held at the end of inspiration and the period of breath-holding could occupy 60% of the entire respiratory cycle. Breath-holding periods interposed between normal ventilatory cycles have also been described in the Domestic Duck (*Anas platyrhynchos*)[10] and the Flamingo (*Phoenicopterus ruber*)[11] and may, according to Bech et al.,[11] be a feature common to the larger species. The practice appears to have no significance in relation to lung aeration but it may offer a positive advantage in that it provides the possibility to increase minute ventilation simply by increasing the rate of breathing, at the expense of the breath-holding period, without altering the depth or duration of individual breaths.

Thermal panting involves a very large increase in respiratory rate. According to Calder and King[12] the increased rate averages 15.7 times the resting value, but recorded increases vary from 9 times in the Ostrich[13] to 35 times in the Rock Partridge (*Alectoris chukar*).[14] Other values include a 19-fold increase in Domestic Fowl,[15] 22- to 23-fold increase in the Flamingo,[11] and a 29-fold increase in the Mute Swan.[16]

III. AIR FLOW IN THE LUNG/AIR SAC SYSTEM

A. Air Flow Pattern in Resting Conditions

Detailed accounts of the structure of the lung/air sac system have previously been published, and only those features necessary for an understanding of the present discussion are dealt with here. The lungs are relatively immobile structures situated in the dorsal thoracic cavity, their external surfaces being deeply indented by the ribs (Figures 5 and 6). Each of the mesobronchi arising from the trachea passes through the length of the lung in the form of a drawn out S shape, and tapers gradually towards its terminal connection to the abdominal air sac. The ventrobronchi, arising from the cranial end of the mesobronchus, connect to the dorsobronchi, arising from the caudal end of the mesobronchus, via the parabronchi, arranged in a series of arcades (Figures 7 through 9). Duncker[17] describes this system as the paleopulmo, which constitutes the entire lung in phylogenetically primitive forms such as Emu (*Dromaius novaehollandiae*), Storks, and Penguins. In more advanced forms, such as the songbirds and gamebirds, Duncker identifies an additional area of parabronchi, the neopulmo, which connects the dorsobronchi and the caudal region of the mesobronchus directly to the abdominal and caudal thoracic air sacs. Duncker surmised on morphological grounds that most of the gas exchange in the resting bird occurs in this restricted area of parabronchi, whilst the paleopulmo becomes better aerated during hyperventilation, as during exercise.

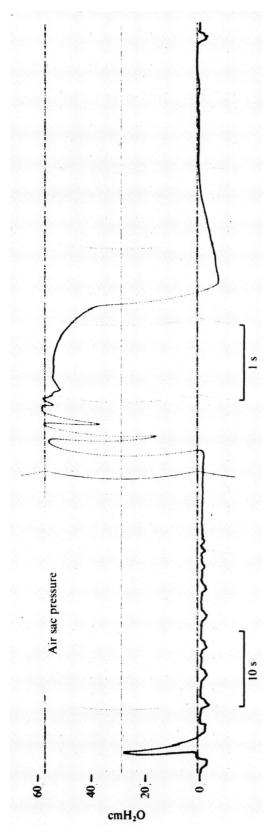

FIGURE 4.   Original recording of air sac pressure during a sequence of normal breaths, followed by a crow in a Domestic Cock. Note differing time scales.

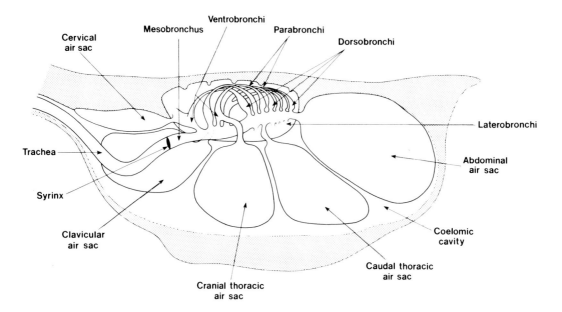

FIGURE 5.   Diagram of the lung/air sac system of the Goose.

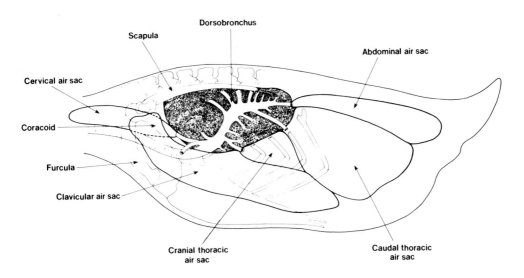

FIGURE 6.   Diagram of the lung/air sac system of a Goose showing relationships with the pectoral girdle, sternum, and ribs.

The precise route taken by the respired gas under the action of the expanding and contracting air sacs has been disputed since the earliest pioneering work of Soum.[18] It is to Brandes[19,20] and Bethe[21] that we owe the most original contribution to the solution to this problem since they first proposed the concept of a unidirectional pattern of air flow through the lung during both phases of respiration. The direction was from the dorsobronchi, across the parabronchi and towards the ventrobronchi. Subsequently several authors claimed to have located anatomical valves that were responsible for the rectification of air flow,[22-26] but the evidence was not convincing and Dotterweich[27] revised an earlier opinion in the light of new experiments carried out on glass models of the lung. He made the novel suggestion that air flow was controlled not by anatomical but by aerodynamic valves, the

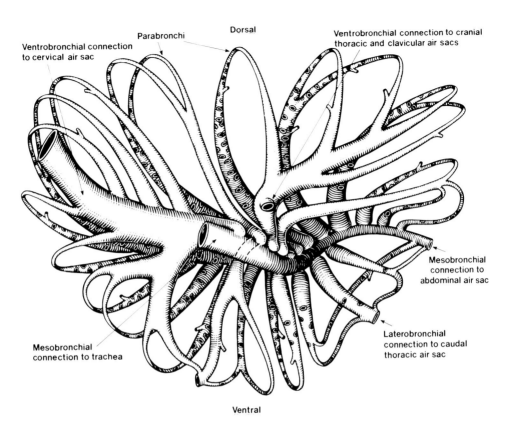

FIGURE 7.   Medial view of the right lung of a Goose drawn from rubber latex casts. Most of the parabronchi have been excluded and only their connections to the secondary bronchi are indicated.

operation of which depended on fluid forces generated within the mesobronchus and secondary bronchi.

Dotterweich's models were only crude representations of the lung, but Hazelhoff[28,29] devised more realistic models and supplemented these with experiments carried out on the lung/air sac system of dead birds. Thus he was able to refine the aerodynamic valve hypothesis and laid down the main ideas which underlie present understanding of the subject. Hazelhoff duplicated the action of the caudal air sacs in dead birds by injecting a stream of air laden with charcoal dust into the sacs and out of the trachea. The stream became deposited in the caudal part of the mesobronchus and entrances to the dorsobronchi. When a similar stream was led into the trachea and out of the caudal air sacs, representing inspiration, the dorsobronchi again became heavily impregnated with dust. Hazelhoff concluded that aerodynamic forces generated inside the caudal part of the mesobronchus must have channelled the air into the dorsobronchi during both phases of respiration, thereby establishing a circulation in the direction mesobronchus → dorsobronchi → parabronchi → ventrobronchi → mesobronchus (the Hazelhoff "loop", Figure 10). The channelling was assisted by two factors: (1) a "guiding dam" or lip on the cranial border of the laterobronchus which connects the caudal thoracic air sac to the mesobronchus; and (2) the acute angle of insertion of this laterobronchus into the mesobronchus, which helped to direct air across the mesobronchus from the laterobronchus to the orifices of the dorsobronchi. Finally, Hazelhoff injected the entire lung air sac system with starch suspension, attached a syringe to the trachea to simulate respiratory movements, and was able to see a stream of granules flowing through the parabronchi lying on the surface of the lung, and traveling in a caudocranial direction during both phases of simulated breathing.

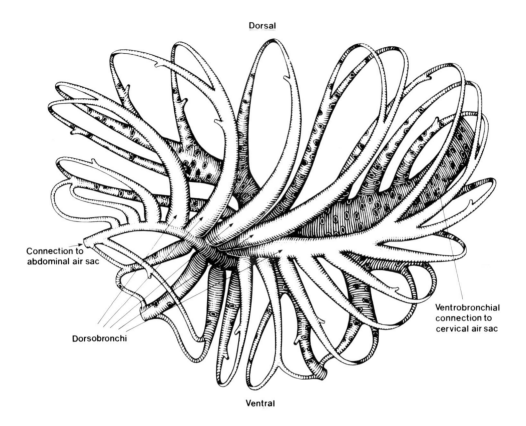

Dorsal

Connection to
abdominal air sac

Dorsobronchi

Ventral

Ventrobronchial
connection to
cervical air sac

FIGURE 8.   Lateral view of the right lung of a Goose.

Using a variety of specially designed flow meters inserted directly into the larger bronchi of the lungs of living birds, Brackenbury,[30] using geese, and Bretz and Schmidt-Nielsen[31] and Scheid and Piiper,[32] both using ducks, were able to confirm the presence of a unidirectional flow of air from the mesobronchus into the dorsobronchi during both phases of respiration (Figures 11 and 12). It was not possible technically to monitor parabronchial air flow but it could be inferred that air must also flow across the parabronchi towards the ventrobronchi.

B. Determinants of Intrapulmonary Air Flow Pattern
1. Evidence from Direct Flow Measurement

Hazelhoff's scheme attributed the intrapulmonary air circulation entirely to the action of the caudal air sacs since the cranial group of sacs was not represented in his models. Aeration of the paleopulmo therefore depended on the operation of the "Hazelhoff loop" which recirculated air through the lung (Figure 10). Recent evidence, however, has thrown doubt on the existence of such a loop. Bretz and Schmidt-Nielsen[31] showed that air flow through both the mesobronchus and the ventrobronchi was not unidirectional, but bidirectional during normal respiration. Scheid et al.[33] perfused fixed duck lung preparations with a reciprocating pump and also found bidirectional flow in the ventrobronchi. Brackenbury[34] simulated the actions of the cranial and caudal groups of air sacs using a unidirectional ventilation technique with anesthetized Geese (*Anser anser*). Thus air led into the trachea and out of a particular air sac represented inspiration by that air sac and vice versa. Air flow was monitored in the dorsobronchi. In the case of the cranial air sacs, simulation of both inspiration and expiration resulted in unidirectional air flow in the dorsobronchi, as occurs during normal respiration.

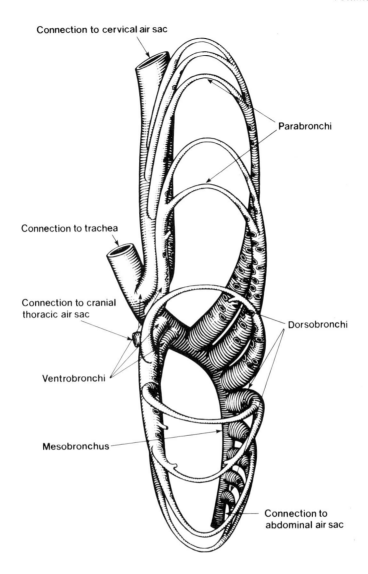

Connection to cervical air sac

Parabronchi

Connection to trachea

Connection to cranial
thoracic air sac

Dorsobronchi

Ventrobronchi

Mesobronchus

Connection to
abdominal air sac

FIGURE 9.   Dorsal view of the right lung of a Goose.

In the case of the caudal sacs, expiration produced a flow of air from the mesobronchus
into the dorsobronchi, as during normal expiration (Figures 13 and 14), but the direction of
air flow in the dorsobronchi resulting from simulated inspiration was dependent on the flow
velocity of the airstream passing into the sac (Figure 15). At low flow rates, such as those
that would be expected during normal breathing at rest, air flowed from the dorsobronchi
into the mesobronchus; i.e., in the opposite direction to that which occurs during normal
inspiration. If the flow rate to the caudal air sacs was increased, however, the dorsobronchial
flow eventually reversed and came to resemble the situation in normal inspiration. These
experiments therefore suggest that the Hazelhoff model accurately portrays the rôle of the
caudal sacs during expiration, but must be qualified as far as inspiration is concerned. During
normal breathing the inherent tendency of the caudal sacs appears to be to draw air into the
ventrobronchi and across the parabronchi towards the dorsobronchi, but this action is masked
by the stronger pull exerted by the cranial sacs which causes air to be drawn into the
dorsobronchi from the caudal end of the mesobronchus. The aeration of the paleopulmo

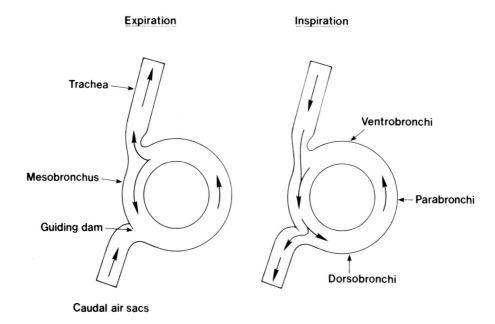

FIGURE 10.   Diagram of Hazelhoff's scheme of air flow pattern in the avian lung.

during inspiration in resting conditions is principally due to the expansion of the cranial sacs, the caudal sacs simply charging with fresh air drawn directly from the mesobronchus. Only at higher respiratory flow rates, such as those that would be associated with exercise hyperpnea, do the independent actions of the cranial and caudal groups of air sacs synchronize to reinforce the entry of air into the dorsobronchi from the mesobronchus.

The foregoing analysis is in keeping with the view that the cranial air sacs behave during inspiration as an aspiratory pump drawing stale air from the parabronchi, which is replaced by a stream of fresh air entering from the mesobronchus. Figure 16 illustrates an experiment which demonstrates the interaction between the cranial and caudal groups of air sacs. First, an airstream (A) was drawn out of the caudal sacs into the atmosphere in order to establish a current from the dorsobronchi into the caudal end of the mesobronchus. Next, a second airstream (B) was drawn from the cranial sacs at a steadily increasing rate. This second stream resulted in a progressive reduction in dorsobronchial flow and eventually a reversal so that air was finally drawn into the dorsobronchi. This experiment illustrates a principle of air flow superposition which probably operates also during normal respiration. The greater aspiratory power of the cranial sacs, drawn open by the expanding but rigid walls of the rib cage, draws air into the dorsobronchi from the caudal end of the mesobronchus, at the expense of the relatively weak tendency of the caudal sacs to draw air out of the dorsobronchi into the mesobronchus. The caudal air sacs, unlike the cranial group, are mainly enclosed by the relatively flexible abdominal walls (Figures 1 and 6) and therefore their aspiratory power is much less. During expiration, the role of the caudal sacs is reversed, since the powerful squeezing action of the abdominal muscles then exerts a dominant effect on intrapulmonary air flow pattern.

One of the most puzzling problems is to explain the mechanism which causes the bulk of the air coming into the mesobronchus during inspiration to be shunted past the ventrobronchial orifices which connect directly with the cranial air sacs (Figures 7 through 9 and 13) and which would seem to present a pathway of low resistance. Molony et al.[7] have shown that the flow resistance between the ventrobronchial orifices and the cranial air sacs is in fact greater than that between the dorsobronchi and the cranial air sacs and they suggested

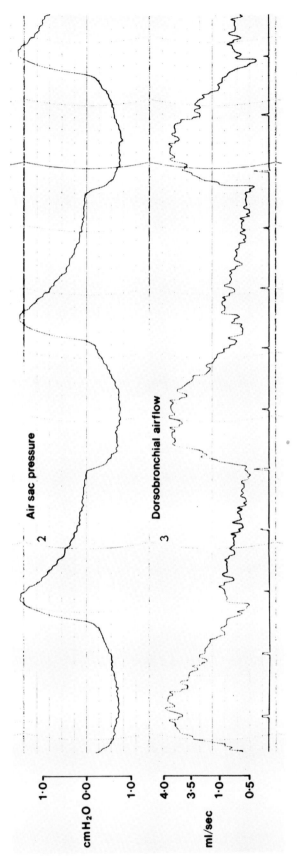

FIGURE 11.   Original recording of air sac pressure and dorsobronchial air flow during normal respiration in a Goose.   Displacements above the zero pressure axis represent expiration.   Dorsobronchial air flow was in the direction mesobronchus → dorsobronchus during both phases of respiration.

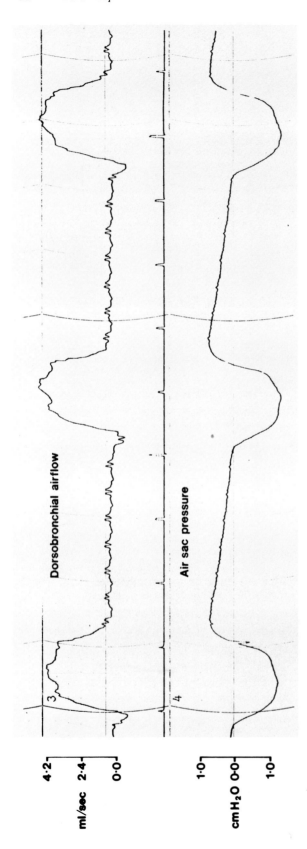

FIGURE 12.   Original recording of dorsobronchial air flow and air sac pressure during normal respiration in a Goose. Note that in this animal there was negligible air flow in the dorsobronchus during expiration. This was probably due to the fact that the bird was lying in the supine position and the abdominal viscera may have collapsed the abdominal air sacs. Inspiratory air flow through the lung, brought about by the cranial air sacs, was not affected.

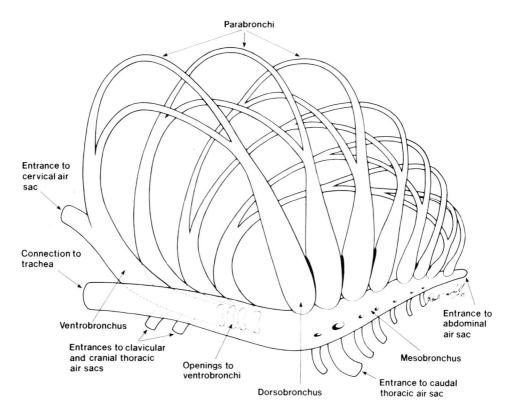

FIGURE 13.   Diagrammatic interpretation of the bronchial structure of the lung upon which Figures 14 through 16 are based.

that this difference might form part of the aerodynamic valving mechanism that seems to determine the unidirectional air flow pattern. They also found that the resistance of the ventrobronchial orifices was susceptible to alterations in intrapulmonary P_{CO_2} providing a potential basis for alterations in airway resistance during the course of the respiratory cycle. In practice, however, this attractive hypothesis does not appear to be the case since, at least according to the radiographic studies of Jones et al.,[35] there is no variation in the caliber of the ventrobronchial orifices during normal breathing. An alternative, mechanical explanation for the routing of air past the ventrobronchial orifices lies in the suggestion[6] that, owing to the acute cranial angle of insertion of the ventrobronchi on to the mesobronchus (Figure 13), air flowing along the mesobronchus from the trachea is, so to speak, "reluctant" to turn the corner into the ventrobronchi. Given that air destined for the expanding cranial air sacs is thus prevented from entering via the ventrobronchi, it must therefore enter via the only remaining route, namely, the dorsobronchi.

2. Evidence from Gas Analysis

Early analyses of the gas composition within various parts of the lung/air sac system showed a pronounced difference between the cranial group of air sacs attached to the ventrobronchi at the cranial end of the mesobronchus, and the caudal air sacs connected to the caudal end of the mesobronchus (Figures 5, and 7 through 9). The concentration of O_2 was 2 to 4% higher and that of CO_2 some 2 to 4% lower in the caudal than in the cranial group.[18,25,36,37] More recent studies employing automatic gas analyzers have confirmed these findings.[3,38-41] Taken together with the existing evidence from direct flow recordings, the distribution of gas compositions between the cranial and caudal air sacs is consistent with

<u>Undirectional airflow into caudal air sacs and out of trachea</u>

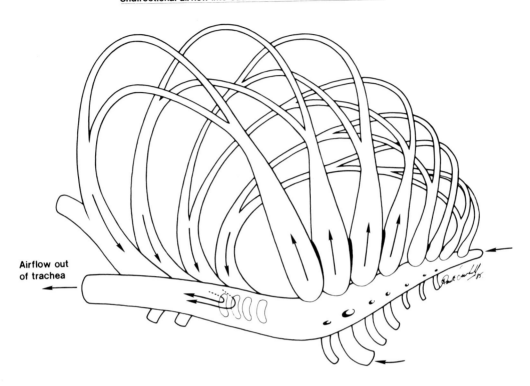

Airflow out
of trachea

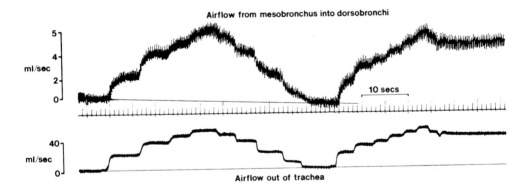

FIGURE 14. Dorsobronchial air flow response to simulated expiration by the caudal air sacs. The bird (a Goose) was unidirectionally ventilated by driving an airstream into the caudal thoracic and abdominal air sacs and out of the trachea, as shown in the upper diagram. The airstream bypassed the cranial air sacs which therefore played no part in ventilation. The lower traces show that stepped increases in the supply stream resulted in corresponding increases in airflow from the mesobronchus into the dorsobronchi.

the following interpretation. During inspiration, the caudal air sacs inspire a mixture of end-expiratory gas and fresh air from the trachea and mesobronchus and this is stored throughout the period of inhalation. At the same time the expansion of the cranial sacs draws stale air out of the parabronchi of the paleopulmo and this is replaced by fresh air drawn in via the dorsobronchial orifices. During the ensuing expiration, the relatively fresh gas stored in the caudal sacs is injected into the caudal end of the mesobronchus and most of it enters the

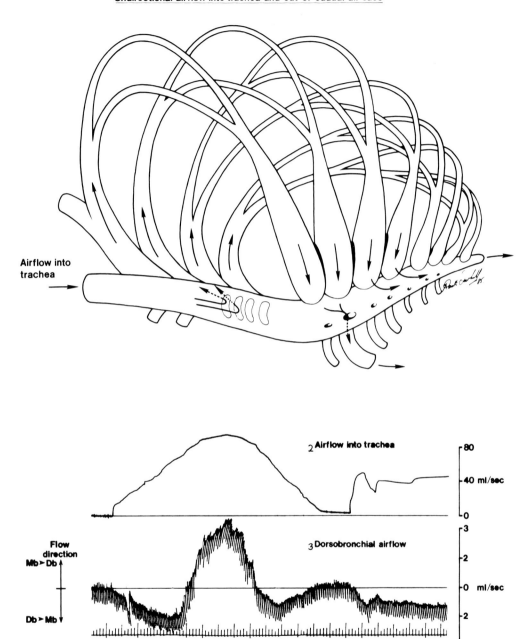

FIGURE 15. Dorsobronchial air flow response to simulated inspiration by the caudal air sacs. A stream of air was driven into the trachea and out of the caudal air sacs, which were opened to the atmosphere, as indicated in the upper diagram. The tracheal air flow rate was steadily increased from zero to a maximum, then back to zero. At relatively low tracheal flow rates, air flowed into the ventrobronchi, across the parabronchi, and out of the dorsobronchi, as shown by the arrows in the diagram. As the tracheal flow increased, air flow through the dorsobronchi ceased, then reversed in direction at the higher tracheal flow rates.

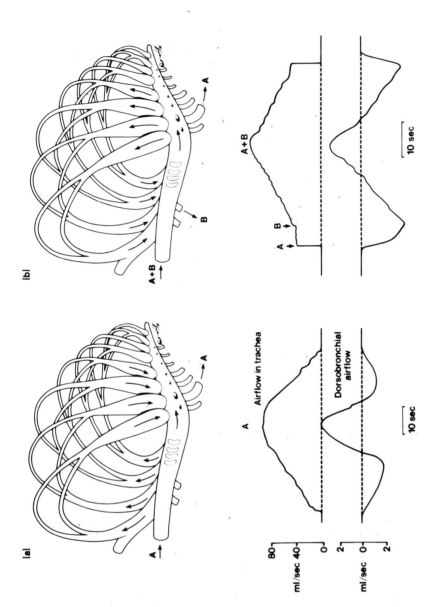

FIGURE 16.　Two different experimental situations which produce reversals of dorsobronchial air flow in the goose lung. (a) is taken from Figure 15. In (b) a unidirectional airstream (A) was led into the trachea and out of the caudal thoracic sac. This established a flow from the dorsobronchi into the caudal end of the mesobronchus. Ten seconds later a second airstream (B) was drawn out of the cranial thoracic air sac at a steadily increasing rate. This caused air flow in the dorsobronchus to diminish and eventually reverse in direction, as shown by the arrows in the upper diagram.

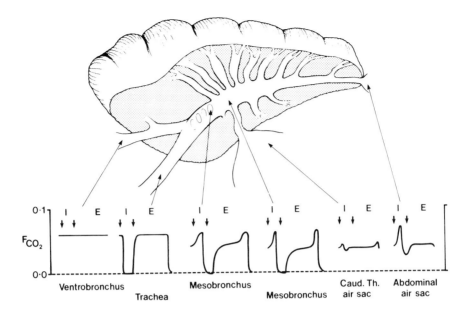

FIGURE 17. F_{CO_2} profiles at various points within the lung/air sac system of duck during normal respiration. The interval between the vertical arrows, marked I, represents inspiration. The period following the second arrow in each breath, marked E, represents expiration. (From Powell, F. L., Geiser, J., Gratz, R. K., and Scheid, P., *Respir. Physiol.*, 44, 195, 1981. With permission.)

dorsobronchi and from there aerates the parabronchi for a second time. Finally, stale air from both the parabronchi and from the collapsing cranial sacs leaves the lung via the ventrobronchi. Here the stale air stream joins with any gas that has leaked along the mesobronchus from the caudal air sacs and the two streams leave via the trachea.

The most thorough examination of gas compositional changes within the lung/air sac system during single respiratory cycles is that carried out by Powell et al.[42] A small cannula was introduced into the mesobronchus, a ventrobronchus, or a dorsobronchus and connected to a mass spectrometer for continuous gas analysis. Within the cranial end of the mesobronchus the expired gas showed a sustained F_{CO_2} plateau (Figure 17). Advancing the cannula along the mesobronchus showed a gradual decline in the height of the end-expired plateau and the maximum F_{CO_2} was registered at the beginning of inspiration when end-expired gas was reinhaled from the trachea. The F_{CO_2} of gas measured in the mesobronchus at the level of the ventrobronchial orifices was significantly higher than that measured at the level of the dorsobronchial orifices. These observations are consistent with the idea that relatively fresh gas exhaled from the caudal sacs enters the dorsobronchi, and that the gas leaving the ventrobronchi and entering the cranial end of the mesobronchus consists of stale air derived both from the cranial air sacs and from the parabronchi. It also supports the view that stale air leaving the lung via the ventrobronchi does not recirculate back along the mesobronchus via the ''Hazelhoff loop''. Powell et al. also found that during inspiration the gas composition of air in the mesobronchus just caudal to the ventrobronchial openings was the same as that of inspired atmospheric air, providing further evidence of the absence of a recurrent flow of stale air along the mesobronchus. Finally, it was shown that the F_{CO_2} along the length of a ventrobronchus was constant throughout the respiratory cycle (Figure 17, left hand side), indicating that inspired air could not have entered the ventrobronchial orifices. This reinforced the idea that an aerodynamic valve exists at the ventrobronchial orifices preventing the entrance of fresh air during inspiration.

C. Gas Flow in the Neopulmo

Although the caudal air sacs receive a stream of fresh air from the mesobronchus during inspiration, their resting P_{CO_2} is nevertheless considerably greater than zero, measuring between 14 and 28 torr according to different authors. Piiper[43] reviewed the possible sources of caudal sac CO_2 and listed, in ascending order of importance, (1) recirculation of gas via the "Hazelhoff loop"; (2) gas exchange in the neopulmo; and (3) reinhalation of end-expired gas from the trachea and mesobronchus. From the discussion in the preceding section it appears that the first factor is not important, while, according to Piiper, reinhalation of dead-space gas probably accounts for 70% of the caudal sac CO_2, leaving 30% to be accounted for by gas exchange in the neopulmo.

Experimental evidence for gas flow in the neopulmo is sparse. Jammes and Bouverot,[40] in a study of breath-to-breath recordings of P_{CO_2} changes in the dorsobronchi of awake Pekin Ducks (*Anas platyrhynchos*), found that at the start of inspiration P_{CO_2} rose to 37 torr as end-expired gas entered from the mesobronchus, then fell to 7 torr as fresh air arrived. During expiration dorsobronchial P_{CO_2} rose to 27 torr and was maintained at this level until the start of the next inspiration. Most of the increased P_{CO_2} must have been due to the influx of gas from the caudal sacs but since the P_{CO_2} of the latter was only 17 to 20 torr, CO_2 must also have been added to the gas on its way from the caudal sacs, presumably as a result of passage through the neopulmo. However, these results were not supported by the data of Powell et al.[42] which showed dorsobronchial P_{CO_2} rising to an expired value that was the same as caudal sac P_{CO_2}. They suggested that the result obtained by Jammes and Bouverot might have been influenced by the high sampling rate used in their experiments. Comparison of dorsobronchial and caudal sac P_{CO_2} can also be made difficult by the fact that, according to Torre-Bueno et al.,[44] complete mixing between inspired and residual gas does not take place during a single breath.

D. Composition of End-Expiratory and Cranial Air Sac Gases

Cohn and Shannon,[3] Vos,[26] Piiper et al.,[38] and Bouverot and Dejours[39] all found that the composition of end-expired gas was similar to that of the cranial air sacs, the discrepancy being less than 5 torr. Complete identity between the two would only be expected if the process of air flow rectification within the paleopulmo was 100% effective. This latter would require that (1) none of the inspired gas enters the cranial sacs via their direct ventrobronchial connections, and (2) all the expired gas leaving the caudal sacs enters the dorsobronchi, none of it leaking forward along the mesobronchus. In these circumstances, since all the inspired gas must have undergone exchange in the parabronchi, the compositions of end-expired, end-parabronchial, and cranial air sac gases would be identical. Cranial air sac gas would then be the equivalent of alveolar gas in the mammalian lung. Since in practice end-expired P_{CO_2} is somewhat lower than that in the cranial sacs, it is likely that a fraction of the caudal sac gas does leak along the mesobronchus during expiration. The direct recordings of Bretz and Schmidt-Nielsen[31] support this view.

IV. VENTILATION AND RESPIRATORY GASES DURING THERMAL PANTING

The only direct recordings of intrapulmonary air flow during panting are those of Bretz and Schmidt-Nielsen[31] whose data showed that the unidirectional pattern remained unchanged. Thermal panting involves very large increases in ventilation of the lung/air sac system, without corresponding increases in the rate of metabolic CO_2 production, despite which the majority of species investigated show only a mild respiratory alkalosis and drops in arterial and intrapulmonary P_{CO_2} of only a few torr[10,11,14-16,45-48] (Figure 18). In all these cases, the birds experienced only moderate thermal stress and displayed a typical pattern of

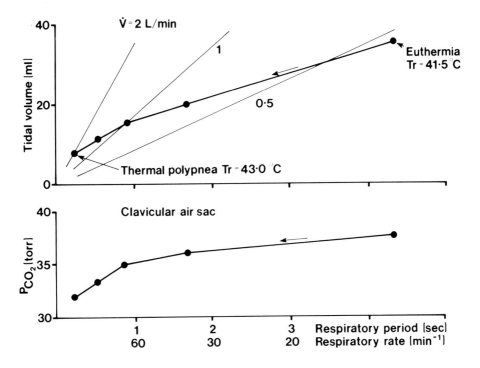

FIGURE 18. Changes in ventilatory characteristics and in clavicular air sac P_{CO_2} during the development of thermal polypnea in Domestic Fowl. At the start of the experiment environmental temperature was 18 to 20°C. The birds were then subjected to an increased environmental temperature (30 to 35°C) for approximately 90 min. The data points represent mean values recorded at different times during the transition towards polypneic breathing, which is indicated by the arrows. Tr, rectal temperature.

polypneic breathing. Other workers[49,50] have found much greater drops in P_{CO_2} but as Bech et al.[11] observe, in such cases the heat stress to which the birds were exposed was probably sufficiently severe to lead to a breakdown of normal thermoregulatory mechanisms.

In order to account for the absence of severe alkalosis during thermal hyperventilation some authors have advocated an intrapulmonary shunt mechanism which channels excess ventilation away from the parabronchi. Such a mechanism, based on muscular valves, was first suggested by Zeuthen[51] and could, in theory at least, be based on the contraction of smooth-muscle sphincters within the dorsobronchi, ventrobronchi, or parabronchi. King and Cowie,[52] for instance, demonstrated that stimulation of the bronchial smooth muscle could lead to airway constriction, but there is still no direct evidence for the operation of anatomical valves in the lung, either during normal breathing or during panting. Moreover, many species have evolved ventilatory strategies which avoid the necessity for any such valvular mechanisms. In Flamingo,[11] Swan,[16] Domestic Fowl,[15] and Pigeon (*Columba livia*),[47] it has been shown that the great reduction in tidal volume that occurs during polypnea is sufficient to confine most of the excess ventilation to the anatomical dead space so that the bulk of the respired air consists of end-expired gas shunted backwards and forwards between the trachea and the lung/air sac system. In heat-stressed Fowl the tidal volume was reduced to only 25% of its normal value and was only 2 mℓ greater than the tracheal volume (6 mℓ). As a result, the effective parabronchial ventilation rose by only 25% compared to an overall fourfold increase in ventilation. Figure 19 shows how successful this strategy is in accurately regulating lung ventilation over a large range of degrees of thermal stress in Pigeon and Pekin Duck.

The Ostrich, however, appears to employ a completely different strategy during hyperthermia. At environmental temperatures of 35 to 45°C, thermal hyperventilation involved a

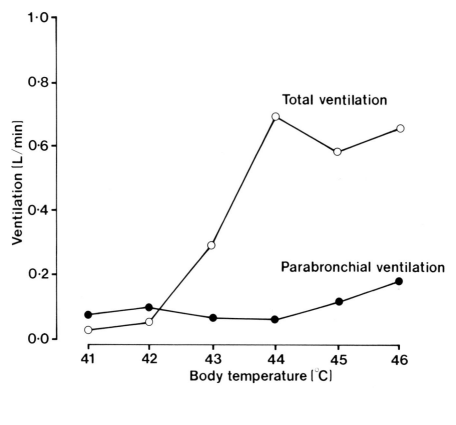

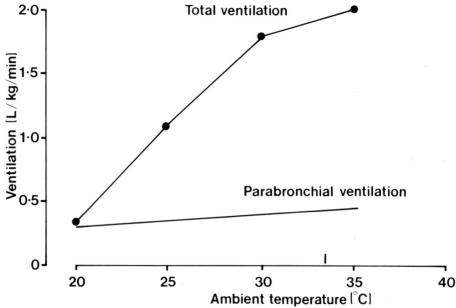

FIGURE 19. Comparison of total ventilation and calculated parabronchial ventilation at different body temperatures in the Pigeon, upper trace (from Bernstein and Samaniego[47]) and at different environmental temperatures in the Pekin Duck, lower trace (from Bouverot et al.[10]).

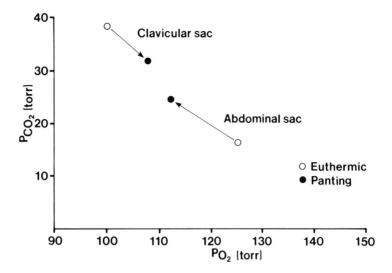

FIGURE 20. P_{O_2} vs. P_{CO_2} diagram of clavicular and abdominal air sac gas composition during normal breathing and thermal panting. (Data from Gleeson and Brackenbury[15]).

seven- to tenfold increase in respiratory rate but in addition a doubling of tidal volume.[53] This meant a 16-fold increase in ventilation of the lung/air sac system caudal to the tracheal dead space. Despite this increase, mean arterial P_{CO_2} and pH did not alter, a result confirming the earlier report by Schmidt-Nielsen et al.[54] The latter authors had, however, found very large drops in cranial and caudal sac P_{CO_2}. These apparently contradictory results could be made compatible if it were assumed, as Jones[53] suggested, that air was somehow shunted past the orifices of the dorsobronchi, thereby avoiding entry to the paleopulmonic parabronchi. Thus air would be forced to pass between the air sacs and the mesobronchus by the direct secondary bronchial connections. It has been estimated that the Reynolds number of the air flow at the base of the trachea in the Ostrich rises from 450 to 1100 at rest to about 10^4 during panting,[54] and turbulence may assist in maintaining a linear flow of air past the dorsobronchial orifices. Jones[53] also examined the possibility that the absence of alkalosis could be due to the shunting of blood away from the lung during panting, thereby creating a severe ventilation/perfusion imbalance, the logical consequence of which could be arterial hypoxemia. In the Ostrich, the blood flow distribution to the lung was only slightly different in panting and nonpanting conditions, but it remains possible that such a change in the ventilation/perfusion ratio could explain the curious situation in the panting Emu[55] which showed a 3-torr drop in arterial P_{CO_2}, suggestive of lung hyperventilation, with a 15-torr drop in arterial P_{O_2} suggestive of lung hypoventilation.

Changes in the gas composition of the air sacs of the panting Fowl are markedly different from those described in the Ostrich, and this may reflect the fundamentally different ventilatory strategies. Mean P_{CO_2} of the cranial sacs decreases while at the same time the P_{CO_2} of the caudal sacs increases, with the result that the gas composition throughout the lung/air sac system becomes almost uniform[15] (Figure 20). Close examination of the caudal sac gas shows that its instantaneous composition varies in a cyclical fashion in phase with changes in the pattern of breathing (Figure 21). During moderate panting, breathing consists of alternating periods of rapid, shallow polypnea, interrupted by brief periods of slower, deeper breathing. During the polypneic sessions stale air accumulates within the caudal air sacs and this is then flushed out during the periods of deeper breathing. This series of events results in regular variations in the rate of gas exchange measured at the mouth (Figure 22). Possible sources of caudal air sac CO_2 have already been reviewed (Section III.C), making

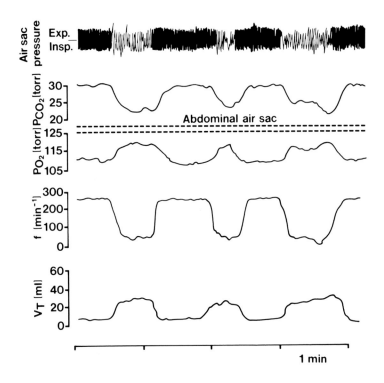

FIGURE 21.   Oscillations in abdominal air sac gas composition related to periodic switching of breathing patterns in the panting Fowl. The air sac pressure trace shows a typical alternation between periods of rapid, shallow breathing, and periods of slower, deeper breathing, as indicated in the two lower traces. During the periods of deeper, slower breathing, stale gas which had accumulated in the caudal sacs throughout the preceding period of polypnea, is "flushed out" and the gas composition of the caudal sacs approaches its normal euthermic value, indicated by the dotted lines. (From Gleeson, M. and Brackenbury, J. H., *Q. J. Exp. Physiol.*, 68, 591, 1983. With permission.)

it likely that such changes are an immediate reflection of the regular alternation in the tidal volume/dead-space ratio.

V. VENTILATION AND RESPIRATORY GASES DURING EXERCISE

The pioneering studies of Hart and Roy[56,57] provided some of the earliest and most valuable information on ventilation in flying birds. The Pigeons used in their experiments were fitted with transducers and telemetric devices which relayed information about respiratory air flow and heart rate during brief periods of free flight. Minute ventilation increased 20-fold and since respiratory rate also increased by the same amount, tidal volume remained unchanged. Lefebvre[58] had earlier shown that the metabolic rate of flying Pigeons increased 8-fold and this led Hart and Roy to conclude that during flight, ventilation must increase 2.5-fold in proportion to metabolic rate. This was consistent with Zeuthen's[51] very early prediction that a Pigeon flying at 50 km · hr^{-1} would double its ventilation in proportion to its metabolic rate in order to evaporate body heat.

All flying birds that have been subsequently studied either in wind tunnels[41,59,60] or during free flight using telemetry[61] increased their respiratory rate, but the change in tidal volume was much more limited varying from zero in the Pigeon to a fourfold increase in the Starling (*Sturnus vulgaris*).[41] However, it is difficult to assess the exact pattern of ventilatory response to flight without taking into account the effects of increased body temperature since active

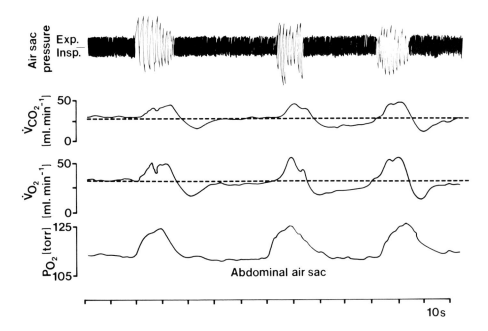

FIGURE 22. Transient variations in O_2 and CO_2 exchange measured at the mouth, caused by the storage and release of stale gas by the caudal air sacs, during thermal hyperventilation. The air sac pressure trace shows polypneic breathing interrupted by three periods of normal breathing during which "flush out" of the caudal sacs takes place. Dotted lines indicate mean values. (From Gleeson, M. and Brackenbury, J. H., *Q. J. Exp. Physiol.*, 68, 591, 1983. With permission.)

birds, like resting birds, develop polypneic breathing when they overheat. It is possible to separate the effects of exercise and temperature by comparing ventilatory responses to work in isothermic and hyperthermic conditions, as was done in Domestic Fowl running on a treadmill.[62-64] When body temperature is held in check by running at reduced ambient temperatures, lung ventilation increases in proportion to gas exchange and there is little change in intrapulmonary or arterial P_{CO_2} over the full range of work loads of which the bird is capable (Figure 23). This precise matching of ventilation and gas exchange is achieved by a ventilatory control strategy that relies principally on increasing respiratory rate in order to meet increased demand for ventilation and permits only relatively small increases in tidal volume. When exercise is performed in hyperthermic conditions, by running the birds at elevated environmental temperatures, the ventilatory strategy must be adapted to cope with the needs of thermoregulation as well as gas exchange and acid-base control. Consequently, the bird hyperventilates but an appropriate adjustment of breathing pattern towards the polypneic mode helps to limit the excess ventilation to the dead space (Figure 24). This strategy is imperfect since it cannot prevent a significant drop in arterial P_{CO_2} from taking place.

In contrast to Domestic Fowl, flying Ravens (*Corvus cryptoleucus*) increased tidal volume as well as respiratory rate in response to an elevation of environmental temperature.[65] It is not known whether this species also avoids alkalosis, for instance by using mechanisms similar to those invoked in the panting Ostrich, or whether it tolerates alkalosis as an acceptable trade-off against overheating. Few data are available on changes that occur in intrapulmonary or arterial P_{CO_2} during exercise in birds. Air sac P_{CO_2} fell during wind-tunnel flight in Starlings[41] and during treadmill exercise in Pekin Duck[66] and Domestic Fowl,[67] and arterial P_{CO_2} dropped by 11 torr during wind-tunnel flight in Pigeon.[60] In all these cases it is likely that lung hyperventilation resulted largely from increased body tem-

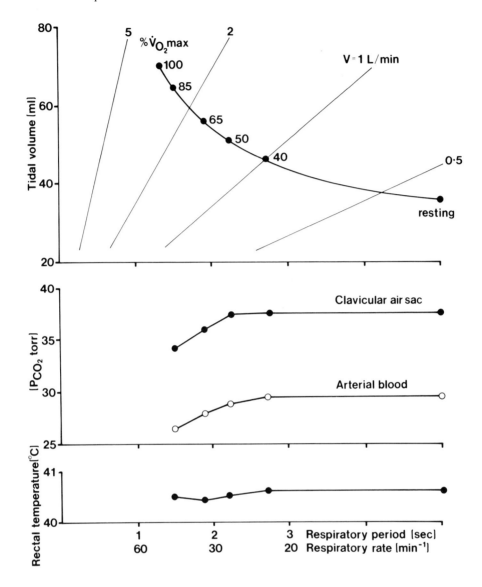

FIGURE 23.   Steady-state ventilatory characteristics, clavicular air sac and arterial P_{CO_2}, and rectal temperature in Domestic Fowl at the end of 10 min of treadmill exercise at different workloads. Exercise took place at reduced environmental temperatures and there was no change in rectal temperature. P_{CO_2} decreased slightly at higher workloads (65 to 100% V_{O_2}) but this could not have been caused by thermal hyperventilation. (Data from Gleeson and Brackenbury[64] and Brackenbury and Gleeson[62].)

perature and, indeed, when Pekin Ducks[68] were run at lowered environmental temperatures the fall in arterial P_{CO_2} was less.

The possible role of spinal thermosensitive neurons in the control of ventilation during exercise has been investigated in cockerels.[69] When these animals ran on a treadmill at an environmental temperature of 9°C, experimental cooling of the spinal cord produced increments of oxygen consumption and ventilation. The increase in minute volume was due to increases in both respiratory rate and tidal volume and the effect was equivalent to that of an increase in exercise intensity. In contrast, spinal cooling during exercise at 34°C reduced both the minute volume and the respiratory rate. Cooling therefore appeared to break the

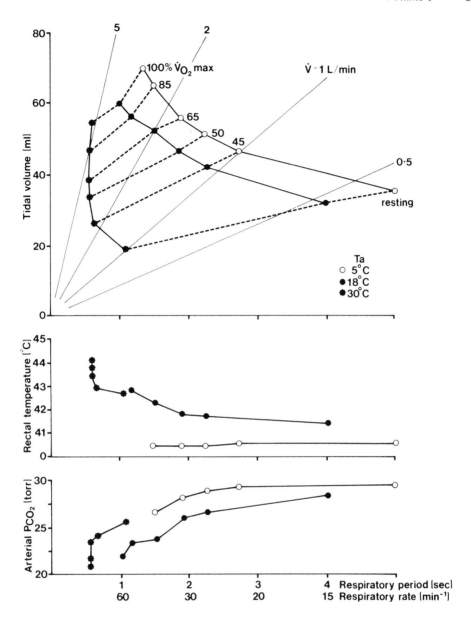

FIGURE 24.   Mean ventilatory characteristics, rectal temperatures, and arterial P_{CO_2} in Domestic Fowl at the end of 10 min of treadmill exercise at different work loads and at ambient temperatures (T_a) of 5, 18, or 30°C. Dotted lines in upper graph join points obtained at equal work loads, and show how increased T_a produced increased respiratory rate but decreased tidal volume. Thermal hyperventilation also led to decreased arterial P_{CO_2}. (From Brackenbury, J. H. and Gleeson, M., *Respir. Physiol.*, 54, 109, 1983. With permission.)

linkage normally operating between the thermoregulatory and respiratory centers. This suggests that spinal thermosensitive neurons may exert a direct effect on motor output from the respiratory center, distinct from secondary effects on respiratory pattern due to altered arterial P_{CO_2}.

Control of breathing pattern in treadmill-exercised Pekin Ducks (*Anas platyrhynchos*), which are not natural runners, appears to differ somewhat from that in Chickens. In this species, increased respiratory rate alone accounted for the hyperpnea of exercise, and tidal volume actually dropped even when running took place in isothermic conditions.[66,68,70] Gleeson et al.[69] have commented that the tracheal cannulation technique employed in the running duck studies might alter the normal pattern of breathing, inhibiting normal changes in tidal volume. It is noteworthy that when Pekin Ducks were exercised in conditions where they also received unidirectional ventilation with CO_2-enriched air, which preserved arterial P_{CO_2} at or slightly above its normal value, both the rate and the depth of breathing increased.[71] A recent study of Tufted Ducks (*Aythya fuligula*) employed a noninvasive mask technique to monitor changes in ventilation and metabolic rate in response to surface swimming exercise.[72] This species is capable of increasing its oxygen consumption during swimming and diving, up to 3.5 times its resting value,[73] which is comparable to the metabolic rate increase observed during treadmill exercise in Pekin Ducks.[70,74] During swimming, most of the ventilatory increase was due to accelerated respiratory rhythm but at the highest work loads tidal volume also increased. In swimming Tufted Duck, running Pekin Duck,[68] and running Chicken,[63] blood lactate increased substantially at higher work loads, a finding implying that the enhancement of tidal volume may be part of a compensatory respiratory response to metabolic acidosis. Additional evidence for the importance of tidal volume as well as respiratory rate in the ventilatory response to exercise has come from studies in which metabolic rate was artificially raised by administration of 2,4-dinitrophenol. In anesthetized, spontaneously breathing Muscovy Ducks (*Cairina moschata*)[75] the increased ventilatory demand was met by increases in both respiratory variables. Some of these birds were hyperthermic and hypocapnic, making it likely that the measured changes in tidal volume were in fact an underestimate of the true, isocapnic response. Gleeson[76] also investigated the effects of injected 2,4-dinitrophenol, as well as of cold exposure, on breathing in unanesthetized Chickens. In these experiments, arterial P_{CO_2} did not alter and the observed changes in respiratory variables (increases in both rate and depth of breathing), were of an identical nature to those produced by isothermic, isocapnic exercise in the fully conscious animal.

The sensitivity of the respiratory pattern generator to alterations in arterial and intrapulmonary P_{CO_2} during exercise is not surprising in view of the role of the specifically CO_2-sensitive intrapulmonary chemoreceptors in the control of avian respiration.[77] However, these receptors do not appear to be directly involved in the ventilatory response to the exercise stimulus, since both Pekin Ducks[78] and Chickens[79] showed the same response to exercise regardless of whether they were breathing air or CO_2-enriched air. There is no direct evidence in birds as to the identity of the factor or factors responsible for exercise hyperpnea, but possible candidates have been reviewed by Kiley and Fedde.[71]

ACKNOWLEDGMENTS

I should like to thank Mr. R. Overhill for the artistic material contained in this chapter. Most of the author's research quoted in the chapter was supported by the Science and Engineering Research Council and the Agricultural and Food Research Council.

REFERENCES

1. **Duncker, H. R.,** General morphological principles of amniotic lungs, in *Respiratory Function in Birds, Adult and Embryonic,* Piiper, J., Ed., Springer-Verlag, Berlin, 1978, 2.
2. **Baer, M.,** Beiträge zur Kenntnis der Anatomie und Physiologie der Atemwerkzeuge bei den Vögeln, *Z. Zool.,* 61, 420, 1896.
3. **Cohn, J. E. and Shannon, R.,** Respiration in unanaesthetized geese, *Respir. Physiol.,* 5, 259, 1968.

4. **Kadono, H., Okada, T., and Ono, K.,** Electromyographic studies on the respiratory muscles of the chicken, *Poult. Sci.,* 42, 121, 1963.
5. **Fedde, M. R., Burger, R. E., and Kitchell, R. L.,** Electromyographic studies on the effects of bodily position and anaesthesia on the activity of the respiratory muscles of the domestic cock, *Poult. Sci.,* 43, 839, 1964.
6. **Brackenbury, J. H.,** Physical determinants of airflow pattern within the avian lung, *Respir. Physiol.,* 15, 384, 1972.
7. **Molony, V., Graf, W., and Scheid, P.,** Effects of CO_2 on pulmonary air flow resistance in the duck, *Respir. Physiol.,* 26, 333, 1976.
8. **Calder, W. A.,** Respiratory and heart rates of birds at rest, *Condor,* 70, 358, 1968.
9. **Bech, C. and Johansen, K.,** Ventilation and gas exchange in the Mute swan, *Cygnus olor, Respir. Physiol.,* 39, 285, 1980.
10. **Bouverot, P., Hildwein, G., and Le Goff, D.,** Evaporative water loss, respiratory pattern, gas exchange and acid-base balance during thermal panting in Pekin ducks under moderate heat exposure, *Respir. Physiol.,* 21, 255, 1974.
11. **Bech, C., Johansen, K., and Maloiy, G. M. O.,** Ventilation and expired gas composition in the flamingo, *Phoenicopterus ruber,* during normal respiration and panting, *Physiol. Zool.,* 52, 313, 1979.
12. **Calder, W. A. and King, J. R.,** Thermal and caloric relations in birds, in *Avian Biology,* Vol. 5, Farner, D. S. and King, J. R., Eds., Academic Press, New York, 1974, 259.
13. **Crawford, E. C. and Schmidt-Nielsen, K.,** Temperature regulation and evaporative cooling in the ostrich, *Am. J. Physiol.,* 212, 347, 1967.
14. **Krausz, S., Bernstein, R., and Marder, J.,** The acid base balance of the rock partridge (*Alectoris Chukar*) exposed to high ambient temperatures, *Comp. Biochem. Physiol.,* 57A, 245, 1977.
15. **Gleeson, M. and Brackenbury, J. H.,** Ventilation, gas exchange and air sac gases during moderate thermal panting in domestic fowl, *Q. J. Exp. Physiol.,* 68, 591, 1983.
16. **Bech, C. and Johansen, K.,** Ventilatory and circulatory responses to hyperthermia in the Mute Swan (*Cygnus olor*), *J. Exp. Biol.,* 88, 195, 1980.
17. **Duncker, H. R.,** The lung-air-sac system of birds, *Ergeb. Anat. Entwicklungsgesch.,* 45(b), 1971.
18. **Soum, M.,** Recherches physiologiques sur l'appareil respiratoire des oiseaux, *Ann. Univ. Lyon,* 28, 236, 1896.
19. **Brandes, G.,** Atmung der Vögel, *Verh. Dtsch. Zool. Ges.,* 28, 57, 1923.
20. **Brandes, G.,** Beobachtungen und Reflexionen über die Atmung der Vögel, *Pflügers Arch. Gesamte Physiol. Menschen Tiere,* 203, 492, 1924.
21. **Bethe, A.,** Atmung: Allgemeines und Vergleichendes, in *Handbuch der normalen und pathologischen Physiologie,* Vol. 2, Bethe, A., Bergmann, G. V., Embden, G., and Ellinger, A., Eds., Springer-Verlag, Berlin, 1925, 1.
22. **Portier, P.,** Sur le rôle physiologique des sacs aériens des oiseaux, *C. R. Soc. Biol.,* 99, 1327, 1928.
23. **Dotterweich, H.,** Versuche über den Weg der Atemluft in der Vogellunge, *Z. Vgl. Physiol.,* 11, 271, 1930.
24. **Dotterweich, A.,** Die Bahnhofstauben und die Frage nach dem Weg der Atemluft, *Zool. Anz.,* 90, 253, 1930.
25. **Dotterweich, H.,** Ein weiterer Beitrag zur Atmungs-physiologie der Vögel, *Z. Vgl. Physiol.,* 18, 803, 1933.
26. **Vos, H. J.,** Über die Wege der Atemluft in der Entenlunge, *Z. Vgl. Physiol.,* 21, 552, 1935.
27. **Dotterweich, H.,** Die Atmung der Vögel, *Z. Vgl. Physiol.,* 23, 744, 1936.
28. **Hazelhoff, E. H.,** Bouw en Functie van de vogellong, *Versl. Gewonne Vergad. Afd. Natuurk., Amsterdam,* 52, 391, 1943.
29. **Hazelhoff, E. H.,** Structure and function of the lung of birds, *Poult. Sci.,* 30, 3, 1951.
30. **Brackenbury, J. H.,** Airflow dynamics in the avian lung as determined by direct and indirect methods, *Respir. Physiol.,* 13, 318, 1971.
31. **Bretz, W. L. and Schmidt-Nielsen, K.,** Bird respiration: flow patterns in the duck lung, *J. Exp. Biol.,* 54, 103, 1971.
32. **Scheid, P. and Piiper, J.,** Direct measurement of the pathway of respired gas in the duck lung, *Respir. Physiol.,* 11, 308, 1971.
33. **Scheid, P., Slama, H., and Piiper, J.,** Mechanisms of unidirectional flow in parabronchi of avian lungs: measurements in duck lung preparations, *Respir. Physiol.,* 14, 83, 1972.
34. **Brackenbury, J. H.,** Corrections to the Hazelhoff model of airflow in the avian lung, *Respir. Physiol.,* 36, 143, 1979.
35. **Jones, J. H., Effmann, E. L., and Schmidt-Nielsen, K.,** Control of air flow in bird lungs: radiographic studies, *Respir. Physiol.,* 45, 121, 1981.
36. **Plantefol, A. and Scharnke, H.,** Contribution a l'étude du rôle des sacs aeriéns dans la respiration des oiseaux, *Ann. Physiol. Physicochim. Biol.,* 10, 83, 1934.

37. **Makowski, J.,** Beitrag zur Klärung des Atmungs-mechanismus der Vögel, *Pflügers Arch. Ges. Physiol.,* 240, 407, 1938.
38. **Piiper, J., Drees, F., and Scheid, P.,** Gas exchange in the domestic fowl during spontaneous breathing and artificial ventilation, *Respir. Physiol.,* 9, 234, 1970.
39. **Bouverot, P. and Dejours, P.,** Pathway of respired gas in the air-sacs-lung apparatus of fowl and ducks, *Respir. Physiol.,* 13, 330, 1971.
40. **Jammes, Y. and Bouverot, P.,** Direct pCO_2 measurements in the dorsobronchial gas of awake Pekin ducks: evidence for a physiological role of the neopulmo in respiratory gas exchange, *Comp. Biochem. Physiol.,* 52A, 635, 1975.
41. **Torre-Bueno, J. R.,** Respiration during flight in birds, in *Respiratory Function in Birds, Adult and Embryonic,* Piiper, J., Ed., Springer-Verlag, Berlin, 1978, 89.
42. **Powell, F. L., Geiser, J., Gratz, R. K., and Scheid, P.,** Airflow in the avian respiratory tract: variations of O_2 and CO_2 concentrations in the bronchi of the duck, *Respir. Physiol.,* 44, 195, 1981.
43. **Piiper, J.,** Origin of carbon dioxide in the caudal air sacs of birds, in *Respiratory Function in Birds, Adult and Embryonic,* Piiper, J., Ed., Springer-Verlag, Berlin, 1978, 148.
44. **Torre-Bueno, J. R., Geiser, J., and Scheid, P.,** Incomplete gas mixing in air sacs of the duck, *Respir. Physiol.,* 42, 109, 1980.
45. **Marder, J., Arad, Z., and Gafni, M.,** The effect of high ambient temperatures on acid-base balance of panting Bedouin Fowl (*Gallus domesticus*), *Physiol. Zool.,* 47, 180, 1974.
46. **Marder, J. and Arad, Z.,** The acid base balance of Abdim's stork (*Sphenorhynchus abdimii*) during thermal panting, *Comp. Biochem. Physiol.,* 51A, 887, 1975.
47. **Bernstein, M. H. and Samaniego, F. C.,** Ventilation and acid-base status during thermal panting in pigeons (*Columba livia*), *Physiol. Zool.,* 54, 308, 1981.
48. **Brackenbury, J. H., Avery, P., and Gleeson, M.,** Effects of temperature on the ventilatory response to inspired CO_2 in unanaesthetized domestic fowl, *Respir. Physiol.,* 49, 235, 1982.
49. **Linsley, J. G. and Burger, R. E.,** Respiratory and cardiovascular responses in the hyperthermic domestic cock, *Poult. Sci.,* 43, 291, 1964.
50. **Mather, F. B., Barnas, G. M., and Burger, R. E.,** The influence of alkalosis on panting, *Comp. Biochem. Physiol.,* 67A, 265, 1980.
51. **Zeuthen, E.,** The ventilation of the respiratory tract in birds, *K. Dan. Vidensk. Kab. Selsk. Biol. Medd.,* 17, 1, 1942.
52. **King, A. S. and Cowie, A. F.,** The functional anatomy of the bronchial muscle of the bird, *J. Anat.,* 105, 323, 1969.
53. **Jones, J. H.,** Pulmonary blood flow distribution in panting ostriches, *J. Appl. Physiol. Respirat. Environ. Exercise Physiol.,* 53, 1411, 1982.
54. **Schmidt-Nielsen, K., Kanwisher, J., Lasiewski, R. C., Cohn, J. E., and Bretz, W. L.,** Temperature regulation and respiration in the ostrich, *Condor,* 71, 341, 1969.
55. **Jones, J. H., Grubb, B., and Schmidt-Nielsen, K.,** Panting in the emu causes arterial hypoxaemia, *Respir. Physiol.,* 54, 189, 1983.
56. **Hart, J. S. and Roy, O. Z.,** Respiratory and cardiac responses to flight in pigeons, *Physiol. Zool.,* 39, 291, 1966.
57. **Hart, J. S. and Roy, O. Z.,** Temperature regulation during flight in pigeons, *Am. J. Physiol.,* 213, 1311, 1967.
58. **Lefebvre, E.,** The use of D_2O^{18} for measuring the energy metabolism in *Columba livia,* at rest and in flight, *Auk,* 81, 403, 1964.
59. **Tucker, V. A.,** Respiratory exchange and evaporative water loss in the flying budgerigar, *J. Exp. Biol.,* 48, 67, 1968.
60. **Butler, P. J., West, N. G., and Jones, D. R.,** Respiratory and cardiovascular responses of the pigeon to sustained level flight in a wind tunnel, *J. Exp. Biol.,* 71, 7, 1977.
61. **Butler, P. J. and Woakes, A. J.,** Heart rate, respiratory frequency and wing beat frequency of free flying Barnacle geese *Branta leucopsis, J. Exp. Biol.,* 85, 213, 1980.
62. **Brackenbury, J. H. and Gleeson, M.,** Effects of PCO_2 on respiratory pattern during thermal and exercise hyperventilation in domestic fowl, *Respir. Physiol.,* 54, 109, 1983.
63. **Gleeson, M. and Brackenbury, J. H.,** Effects of body temperature on ventilation, blood gases and acid-base balance in exercising fowl, *Q. J. Exp. Physiol.,* 69, 61, 1984.
64. **Gleeson, M. and Brackenbury, J. H.,** Respiratory and blood gas responses in exercising birds, *Comp. Biochem. Physiol.,* 76A, 211, 1983.
65. **Hudson, D. M. and Bernstein, M. H.,** Temperature regulation and heat balance in flying white-necked ravens, *Corvus cryptoleucus, J. Exp. Biol.,* 90, 267, 1981.
66. **Kiley, J. P., Kuhlmann, W. D., and Fedde, M. R.,** Respiratory and cardiovascular responses to exercise in the duck, *J. Appl. Physiol Respirat. Environ. Exercise Physiol.,* 47, 827, 1979.

67. **Brackenbury, J. H., Gleeson, M., and Avery, P.,** Effects of sustained running exercise on lung air-sac gas composition and respiratory pattern in domestic fowl, *Comp. Biochem. Physiol.,* 69A, 449, 1981.

68. **Kiley, J. P., Kuhlmann, W. D., and Fedde, M. R.,** Ventilatory and blood gas adjustments in exercising isothermic ducks, *J. Comp. Physiol.,* 147, 107, 1982.

69. **Gleeson, M., Barnas, G. M., and Rautenberg, W.,** Respiratory and cardiovascular responses of the exercising chicken to spinal cord cooling at different ambient temperatures. II. Respiratory responses, *J. Exp. Biol.,* 114, 427, 1985.

70. **Kiley, J. P., Faraci, F. M., and Fedde, M. R.,** Gas exchange during exercise in hypoxic ducks, *Respir. Physiol.,* 59, 105, 1985.

71. **Kiley, J. P. and Fedde, M. R.,** Cardiopulmonary control during exercise in the duck, *J. Appl. Physiol.: Respirat. Environ. Exercise Physiol.,* 55, 1574, 1983.

72. **Woakes, A. J. and Butler, P. J.,** Respiratory, circulatory and metabolic adjustments during swimming in the Tufted duck, *Aythya fuligula, J. Exp. Biol.,* 120, 215, 1986.

73. **Woakes, A. J. and Butler, P. J.,** Swimming and diving in Tufted ducks, *Aythya fuligula,* with particular reference to heart rate and gas exchange, *J. Exp. Biol.,* 107, 311, 1983.

74. **Bech, C. and Nomoto, S.,** Cardiovascular changes associated wtih treadmill running in the Pekin duck, *J. Exp. Biol.,* 97, 345, 1982.

75. **Geiser, J., Gratz, R. K., Hiramoto, T., and Scheid, P.,** Effects of increasing metabolism by 2,4-dinitrophenol on respiration and pulmonary gas exchange in the duck, *Respir. Physiol.,* 57, 1, 1984.

76. **Gleeson, M.,** Respiratory adjustments of the unanaesthetized chicken, *Gallus domesticus,* to elevated metabolism elicited by 2,4-dinitrophenol or cold exposure, *Comp. Biochem. Physiol.,* 83A, 283, 1986.

77. **Bouverot, P.,** Control of breathing in birds as compared with mammals, *Physiol. Rev.,* 58, 604, 1978.

78. **Kiley, J. P. and Fedde, M. R.,** Exercise hyperpnea in the duck without intrapulmonary chemoreceptor involvement, *Respir. Physiol.,* 53, 355, 1983.

79. **Brackenbury, J. H. and Gleeson, M.,** Exercise hyperpnea in birds: evidence against a primary role for PCO_2, *Comp. Biochem. Physiol.,* 83A, 337, 1986.

Chapter 3

PHONATION

Abbot S. Gaunt

TABLE OF CONTENTS

I. INTRODUCTION

Phonation is an important component of avian behavior. Indeed, vocal communication begins prior to hatching and can strongly influence the rate of development.[1] Avian vocal systems are similar to those of mammals and anurans in that sound is produced by an airflow interacting with a modified portion of the ventilatory tract, but they are dissimilar in a variety of other characteristics. The vocal organ, or syrinx, is not associated with the larynx but is a modification of the trachea and/or bronchi. Modulation of evoked sounds does not depend on the resonance properties of the vocal tract. Many birds can produce two harmonically unrelated tones simultaneously, and some can modulate those tones independently.

II. SYRINGEAL STRUCTURE

The best source of descriptions of the external morphology of syringes remains Beddard.[2] Ames[3] presents a thorough description of syringes within the Passeriformes. Histological descriptions of syringes for many species are distributed widely in the literature, but no good summary is readily available. Perhaps the best is Warner's doctoral thesis,[4] of which portions presenting the data for Ducks,[5] Doves,[6] and Oscines[7] have been published. The following description should be sufficient to permit an understanding of the action of a syrinx in avian phonation.

A. Position

The syrinx is situated deep within the interclavicular air sac in the thoracic cavity (Figure 1). In a few birds, notably Goatsuckers (Caprimulgiformes), Cuckoos (Cuculidae), and some Owls (Strigidae), a syrinx may occur in each bronchus. Only the caudal end of the trachea is involved in the suboscine Superfamily Furnaroidea and in Storks (Ciconiidae). In Parrots (Psittaciformes), the syrinx is intermediate between tracheal and tracheobroncheal, containing both tracheal and bronchial elements but having only one, tracheal site for sound production.[8,9] In other birds, the syrinx is at the tracheobronchial junction and lies immediately dorsocraniad of the heart. The dorsal surface of the syrinx is tightly adhered to the esophagus, but all other surfaces are exposed to the contents of the interclavicular air sac. To some extent the designations tracheal and tracheobronchial are artificial. As noted by Ames,[3] the key depends on whether the medial tympanic membranes, which are bronchial, participate in sound production. In Hummingbirds (Trochilidae), the interclavicular air sac extends craniad onto the neck, and the tracheobronchial junction and syrinx are shifted correspondingly.

B. Components

A syrinx is composed of one or more flexible portions and their skeletal supports (Figure 2). The flexible portions are generally termed tympanic membranes, although thicker ones are sometimes called labia. The supporting elements are the tracheal rings, which are usually bony and complete and sometimes have interlocking edges, and the bronchial half-rings, which are usually cartilagenous and have an open side medially. By convention, all supporting elements are numbered from the syrinx, thereby eliminating problems arising from windpipes of different lengths. The first few tracheal rings are often fused to form a tympanum or drum. A triangular pessulus, which may extend dorsoventrally as a strut across the caudal end of the tympanum, often stiffens the medial junction of the bronchi. The pessulus is absent from Doves (Columbiformes), Parrots, Swallows (Hirundinidae), and Tyrant Flycatchers (Tyranidae).

C. Musculature

The syringeal muscles are paired to the right and left sides and are divided into two

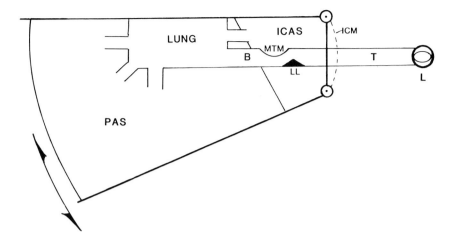

FIGURE 1. A diagrammatic schema of the avian vocal system. The bird's body is shown as a large bellows. Contraction of the abdominal muscles compresses the bellow, or air sacs, and forces air through the syrinx, where it can interact with the lateral and/or medial tympanic membranes. The bore of the syringeal lumen can be adjusted either by the position of the membranes or the insertion of a lateral labium. Abbreviations: B, bronchus; ICAS, interclavicular air sac (which is fused with the anterior thoracic air sacs in oscines); ICM, interclavicular membrane; L, larynx; LL, lateral labium; MTM, medial tympanic membrane; PAS, posterior air sacs (abdominal and posterior thoracic air sacs, and including the anterior thoracic air sacs in those species in which they are not fused to the ICAS); T, trachea. (From Gaunt, A. S. and Gaunt, S. L. L., in *Current Ornithology*, Vol. 2, Johnston, R. F., Ed., Plenum Press, New York, 1985. With permission.)

groups, extrinsic and intrinsic. The extrinsic muscles are the sternotrachealis and tracheolateralis. The former extends from the sternum forward to insert on the trachea about midway between the drum and the interclavicular membrane. Its presumed action is to draw the trachea caudad and relax the syringeal membranes. The tracheolateralis runs along the sides of the trachea from the larynx to the vicinity of the syrinx. In some species it is restricted to the caudal portion of the trachea. It is a presumed antagonist of the sternotrachealis. A third muscle, the cleidohyoideus (= ypsilotrachealis or tracheohyoidius), which in some species extends from the clavicles to the trachea, thence craniad to the hyoid, may also act in concert with the sternotrachealis to draw the trachea caudad.[10-12] With rare exceptions, extrinsic muscles are distributed throughout the class Aves.

Intrinsic muscles, which arise from the trachea and insert on bronchial elements, are confined to the Parrots, Hummingbirds, several families of suboscine Passeriformes, and the songbirds (Oscines). Oscines possess by far the most elaborate syringes (Figure 2), with two extrinsic muscles, four to five (depending on what is counted) intrinsic muscles, a lateral labium and its associated lateral tympanic membrane, and a medial tympanic membrane on each side.

The extrinsic muscles are derived from tracheal muscles, and it is generally agreed that intrinsic muscles arose from the tracheolateralis.[3] In fact, the *bronchotrachealis anticus* and *posticus* of Oscines appear to be little more than continuations of the tracheolateralis. In many nonoscines, including the ratites, the tracheolateralis extends onto the syrinx proper and may even insert onto bronchial elements.[2] As it can contract by sections,[10] it may function as both an extrinsic and an intrinsic muscle in these birds.

The presence of intrinsic muscles appears to be an important precursor to the evolution of learned vocal behavior and large repertoires. However the absence of a strong, or even evident, correlation between the degree of complexity of syringeal structure and vocal abilities suggests that complex syringes evolved under selective pressures for some other biologic role.[13]

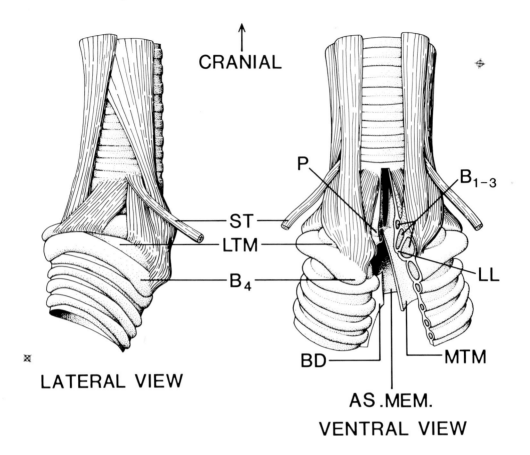

↑
CRANIAL

ST
LTM
B₄

LATERAL VIEW

P
B₁₋₃
LL
BD
MTM
AS.MEM.
VENTRAL VIEW

FIGURE 2.   Lateral and ventral views of the syrinx of a songbird. In the ventral view, a portion of the left bronchus has been removed to show a saggital section. The bronchidesmus (BD), which extends between the median walls of the bronchi, usually just caudal to the MTM, has been cut. The interclavicular air sac extends dorsad between the bronchidesmus and the pessulus (P). Its dorsal wall is visible between the bronchi (AS. MEM.). Except for the sternotrachealis (ST), all the illustrated muscles are intrinsic. The two muscles running craniad on the lateral margins of the trachea will join at about the level of the interclavicular membrane to become the tracheolateralis. This rendition is slightly idealized, but is based on the syrinx of a Steller's Jay, *Cyanocitta stelleri*. Other abbreviations: B_1 through B_4, bronchial bars 1 through 4; LL, lateral labium; LTM, lateral tympanic membrane.

III. NEURAL CONTROL

The syringeal muscles are innervated by branches of the hypoglossal nerve. Crossover of the innervation between the two sides of the syrinx (or trachea) occurs in Chickens,[10] Ducks,[11] and Parrots.[8,14] In songbirds, the innervation is unilateral and ipsilateral, with the left side being dominant.[14-19] Oddly, bilaterally severing the hypoglossals does not necessarily silence a bird, so action of the syringeal muscles is not a necessity for vocalization. Songbird songs are drastically altered, and some hypoglossectomized songbirds may die from asphyxia, although others can survive in the wild and may successfully migrate.[15,16,19-21] In contrast, anesthetized, hypoglossectomized Chickens (*Gallus gallus* = *G. domesticus* of authors) produce almost normal clucks during electrical brain stimulation (EBS).[10]

Because phonation is driven by the ventilatory mechanism, we might expect a close relationship between the neural control of respiration and the neural control of vocalization, but that expectation is met only partially. In a series of studies,[10,22-24] the "Minnesota group" of Peek, Phillips, and Youngren established the presence of a midbrain vocal center that controlled repetitive vocalizations in Chickens. They proposed that a single center controlled both respiratory and ventilatory rhythms. Similar centers have been found in other nonpasserines and in oscines.[25-28] Brackenbury[29] showed that the repetitive calls of Chickens and Domestic Geese (*Anser anser*) occur at the frequencies of thermal panting. Richards[30] obtained clucking sounds synchronized with respiration from Chickens when the panting centers of the brain were electrically stimulated.

More complex vocalizations, especially oscine songs, are controlled from the forebrain via a direct pathway to the hypoglossal nucleus. The neural control of singing, its interrelationship with hormonal control, and relationship to learning have been reviewed recently by Arnold[31] and Nottebohm.[32]

IV. MECHANICS

A. General Principles

In humans[33] and anurans,[34] a repositioning of the laryngeal cartilages interposes the vocal folds into the airstream of the trachea. When subglottal pressure is sufficient, the folds are blown open, whereupon Bernoulli forces, elasticity of the folds, and reduced subglottal pressure restore the folds to their original positions and subglottal pressure again builds. This cycle introduces a series of pulses of air into the vocal tract; i.e., the pharyngeal, nasal, and buccal cavities. The resulting pulse tone has a fundamental frequency that is determined by the rate of pulse generation and a series of harmonics of that fundamental. By adjusting the shapes of the vocal tract, a human establishes a series of resonant filters that damp some frequencies while augmenting others. Different combinations of frequencies produce the different vowel sounds. The pitch of the voice is controlled by adjusting the tension of the vocal folds, which determines the rate of pulse formation. In a similar way, vibrating lips or reeds act as pulse generators to stimulate the resonance properties of various wind instruments. The fundamental frequency of the instrument is determined by the length of the resonating tube.[35] Many early hypotheses of the mechanics of avian phonation (reviewed in Greenewalt[36]) assumed a system similar to that of humans or wind instruments, and much confusion has arisen (and still occurs) from attempts to analogize the avian vocal system with either or both of these resonance-controlled systems. Our present ideas are derived largely from the studies of Greenewalt[36] and Stein.[37]

B. Models of Syringeal Function

The exact nature of the interaction between the syringeal membranes and the airstream remains ambiguous. At least three, not necessarily mutually exclusive, models seem plausible (Figure 3). In the classic model, the syrinx is first relaxed by muscular action. In those birds with only extrinsic muscles, the sternotrachealis is the effector. It may perform a similar role in other birds, but its action could be replaced by activities of the intrinsic muscles.[9,12,38] Bernoulli forces then draw the relaxed membrane into the lumen until it tenses and elastic-restoring forces reverse the movement. Brackenbury[39] observed that a stable balance between Bernoulli forces and membrane elastic forces is unlikely because the former varies linearly, the latter curvilinearly. Thus, a cyclic oscillation essentially normal to the direction of airflow is established. The membrane presents a surface to the airstream and vibrates as such. The surface may be distorted downstream in a manner that permits a series of waves or ripples to translate along the surface in the direction of airflow. Such ripples are often presumed to be responsible for harmonic frequencies.[36,40,41]

A problem with this model is that freely oscillating membranes produce sounds that are rich in overtones at nonharmonic intervals,[35,42] whereas avian phonations are usually composed of single frequencies (whistles) or harmonic tones. It is usually an implicit, and sometimes an explicit, assumption of the classic model that edge effects are negligible or

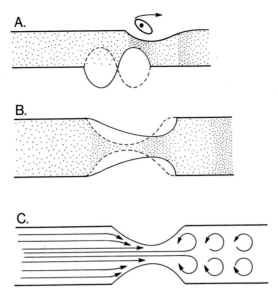

FIGURE 3.   Three models of the actions of syringeal membranes in sound production. (A) The classic model, in which
vibrations of the membranes expand or constrict the diameter of the bronchial passage, thereby rarifying or com-
pressing the air. The diameter of the tube may also be varied
by insertion of the lateral labium opposite the membrane.
(B) Pulse tone model, in which membranes occlude the
passage until blown apart, releasing a pulse of pressure. (C)
A whistle, in which the membranes do not vibrate but rather
provide a flexible zone that can be shaped into a slot. Turbulence produced by air jetting through the slot forms an
aerodynamic sound source. See text. (Modified from Gaunt,
A. S. and Gaunt, S. L. L., in *Current Ornithology*, Vol.
2, Johnston, R. F., Ed., Plenum Press, New York, 1985.
With permission.)

at least evenly distributed. But the medial tympanic membrane in a songbird's syrinx is
supported along its lateral margins by highly elastic, cartilagenous, bronchial half-rings.
Any relaxation that would permit movement into the airstream could occur only along the
caudocranial axis. Further, many of the intrinsic muscles are so arranged that their contraction
will produce forces with outwardly directed components. Thus, while the membrane is
relaxing along a caudocranial axis, tension in the dorsoventral axis will be maintained or
even increased, and the membrane will move into the lumen not as a surface but as a fold
that presents an edge to the airstream. The lateral tympanic membranes in many birds are
so shaped and supported that they also tend to fold inward along an axis rather than bulge
inward as a surface. In these cases, the syringeal membranes begin to resemble human vocal
folds, and sound may be generated, but not modulated, by a similar mechanism. As in the
classical model, pitch (frequency) would be determined by the tension of the fold(s). As
the tension increases, the oscillation would move toward the edge. In the limiting case, only
the edge would vibrate and could be regarded as a string, a mechanism that does produce
harmonics. This folded edge or vocal fold arrangement acts as a pulse generator and represents
the second model.[43]

Models in which vibrating membranes are the sound source are supported by many
observations that the membranes of dissected syringes do oscillate in a sufficient airflow
and, more important, that the oscillations may match the fundamental frequency of the

elicited sound.[44] Of course, injuring the membranes could also prevent them from reshaping to form a whistle. Further, stiffening or otherwise injuring the membranes of living birds prevents phonation.[45-47] Presumably, then, the frequency of the sound is determined by the tension of the membrane, which could be adjusted directly by action of syringeal muscles.

If the folded edges of the membranes approach each other or the opposite wall so as to form a slot or small aperature, and if the vibration of the membranes is minimized, perhaps by strong tension, then conditions may obtain for a third mechanism, a turbulence shedding slot or whistle.[48] This mechanism does not depend on membrane vibration. The vocal folds of freshly dissected human larynges can be drawn into such a slot, and some living humans are capable of glottal whistling.[49] Such a mechanism could account for the pure tones that are the most widely distributed of all avian phonations. The three mechanisms could easily form a continuum, of which most species exploit only a portion. Some species, however, (e.g., many corvids, sturnids, mimids, and psittacids) command the entire range.

C. Modulation and Resonance

Most, if not all, modulations of avian phonations are source generated. Evidence for this hypothesis comes from a variety of sources, many of which were developed and exemplified by Greenewalt.[36] First, there is no correlation between the length of a bird's trachea and the fundamental frequency of its phonations. Assuming that the trachea acts as a tube open at one end, the call of a Spruce Grouse (*Canachites canadensis*) at 85 to 90 Hz would require a tracheal length of 100 cm. Conversely, a trachea of only 10.5 cm would be needed to produce the call of a Whistling Swan (*Cygnus columbianus*) with a fundamental frequency of 840 Hz. Even the inordinately long trachea of a Crane (Gruidae) does not seem to determine the fundamentals of its calls.[36,50] The "breaking of the voice" when the juvenal calls of many birds convert to the adult calls is influenced as much by hormonal state as by tracheal length.[51] Second, analysis of songs that contain glissandi or otherwise exhibit a range of frequencies shows no forbidden frequencies, i.e., frequencies that would be strongly damped by a simple, tubular resonator. Third, the pitch of resonance-controlled phonations, such as human voice, is partially determined by the speed of sound in the resonating chamber, which, in turn, depends on the density of the enclosed fluid medium. Hence, humans breathing a mixture of helium and oxygen speak with high-pitched voices. Birds are much less affected. Those that have whistled songs (no overtones) show no effect; those with many overtones may show some slight shifting, but it is not as dramatic as that of humans.[50,52] The slight shifts that we do see in some calls might be explained by the relatively minor effects of a changed air density on the vibrating membranes.[36] Finally, the presence and independent modulation of two voices (see Section V) would be impossible if both sources were subservient to the resonant properties of a single tube.

Several papers have presented data seemingly at variance with the Greenewalt-Stein Model. Myers[53] reported that the calls of a Rooster increased in pitch if its trachea was surgically shortened. Rüppell[54] elicited sounds by blowing through the dissected syrinx and trachea of a Crane and found that pitch increased as the trachea was shortened. Greenewalt[36] expressed skepticism of the results of experiments with isolated syringes and tracheae because his explanation of the lack of tracheal resonance depends on a specific ratio between tracheal and syringeal bore during phonation, a ratio that may not be achieved in artificial conditions. His doubts seem justified. Gaunt et al.[50] surgically shortened tracheae in live Cranes of several species and determined that, although the voices acquired additional overtones, neither the fundamental nor highest overtones were significantly higher. The change in pitch observed by Myers may have resulted from severing the hypoglossal nerve, which would inactivate the syringeal musculature and change tension relationships of the syrinx.

Sutherland and McChesney[55] reported that the calls of Ross's Goose (*Chen rossii*) were higher pitched than those of the larger Snow Goose (*Chen caeruleans*), and that the harmonics of both calls agreed with the hypothesis of the trachea as a resonating tube open at both ends. However, the differences in pitch can be accounted for as well by the differences in size of the oscillating membranes in the two species.[56]

Although there is little evidence to support tracheal resonance as a determining factor in avian phonation, resonance phenomena may yet play some role. Harris et al.[57] suggest that the trachea, beak, and oral cavity of a rooster may "tune the sound of vocalization . . . to a resonant frequency, which causes the pitch to be more sharply defined". The effect of helium on some whistled songs is to elicit an overtone at or near the frequency expected for the second harmonic. This suggests that the vocal systems of affected birds possess resonance peaks at or near the frequencies of their fundamentals, and that the helium shifts peak sufficiently to activate a formant-like resonance at the second harmonic.[57a,57b] The birds that have been tested are generally small and have high-pitched songs with fundamentals near the range that could be augmented by the resonance of a short trachea. Certainly, if a trachea has a resonance peak near the frequency produced by the sound source, selection for the loudest song with least effort would promote convergence of the two. In this case, tracheal resonances would be weakly coupled as in humans, and the effect of helium would be to shift the resonance peak, or formant, not to change the fundamental. Nontracheal resonances may also be important in some birds.[50]

Greenewalt[36] observed that frequency and amplitude modulations (FM and AM) are frequently linked in avian phonations. In the lower portions of a bird's frequency range, the linkage is direct, but as frequency increases, there comes a point at which the linkage inverts and amplitude decreases with further increases in frequency. He suggested that a relaxed membrane, which would produce low frequencies, moves far into the lumen where its vibrations are constrained by proximity of the opposite wall or membrane. As tension, hence frequency, increases, the membrane is withdrawn from the lumen and the amplitude of the oscillations increases. Eventually, increasing tension damps the oscillations, and amplitude again decreases. However, such spatial constraints are likely to induce nonlinearities leading to rippling (= harmonic?) oscillations rather than simply to reduce amplitude. Hinsch[58] noted that the pattern of linkages suggested a resonating system. He supposed that amplitude rose and fell as the vibratory frequency of the membrane approached or diverged from the resonance frequency of the trachea, but that explanation seems unlikely.

Gaunt and Wells[59] proposed a resonating system involving only membranes and airflow. They suggested that membrane oscillation was driven by periodic disturbances in the airflow, and that amplitude increased as the periodicity of the disturbance approached the resonant frequency of the membrane. The observed rise and fall in amplitude with increasing frequency would occur if either the tension of the membrane were constant as the periodicity of the disturbance increased, or vice versa. Klatt and Stefanski[41] proposed a similar model. This hypothesis leads easily to the notion of a system in which aerodynamic events (whistles) are the source of the sound and the membranes act either as entrained resonators (a driven membrane can produce either pure or harmonic sounds — otherwise radio speakers would not work), or simply as flexible structures used to form a vortex-shedding slot. The frequency of some whistles varies directly with flow rate.[60] As the membranes are withdrawn, the aperture between them increases, thereby decreasing flow rate and lowering the pitch. Beebe[61] and Paulsen[44] observed that the frequency of the sound produced from isolated syringes may drop as membranes are withdrawn from the lumen, i.e., when tension is presumably increasing the membrane-generated sounds should increase in pitch. The pitch of other whistles may be stable over a considerable range of airflow, then suddenly shift as a threshold value is achieved.[62] A sudden change of pitch is characteristic of many avian calls, e.g., the "long calls" of Gulls (Charadriidae). Abs[51] has shown that such shifts can be produced by changes of airflow. If a feedback loop should develop between the rate of vortex shedding and membrane oscillation, then tension of the membrane could determine the frequency of the whistle, and distinctions between sound source and responder would be essentially arbitrary.

Stein[37] showed that many avian calls can be easily interpreted as a carrier frequency affected by one or more modulating frequencies. In particular, many amplitude modulations appear to be relatively slow modulating frequencies acting on high carrier frequencies. Oscillations of the relatively massive lateral labia might produce such effects. Stein also suggested that a link between AM and FM occurred because the mechanics of adjusting the oscillations of the medial tympanic membrane and the lateral labium were linked. Interestingly, Greenewalt[36] felt that the movement of the lateral labium into the lumen would constrain membrane oscillation and could account for those instances in which AM and FM were not linked!

V. MULTIPLE VOICES

Many species with tracheobronchial syringes can produce two harmonically unrelated tones simultaneously. These tones are sometimes detectable on a sound spectrograph,[63] but can be clearly demonstrated with an oscilloscope and narrow bandpass filters. Given that avian phonations are source generated, then it is easy to imagine that one tone is produced by each side of a tracheobronchial syrinx. In Oscines, the two sides are independently controlled and can be independently modulated.[15-19] Hence, an individual can literally duet with itself. This capability is termed the "two-voice" phenomenon.

The presence of three or four voices has been reported for some birds,[64-66] but a mechanism for their production remains obscure, unless we assume that each lateral and medial membrane produces a different sound. However, the lateral membranes of Oscines do not seem to be a sound source.[45] Further, nonharmonic overtones can be produced by a wide variety of means.[35,67] Hence, suggestions of multiple voices should show that each "voice" is independent of the others.

When present, the two voices may be clearly independent or may interact to produce more complex sounds. Two pure tones of slightly different frequencies can produce a single tone with a beat.[37,48] When each side generates an harmonically complex tone, the interaction can be nonlinear and very complex.[67a] The resulting sound may resemble an harmonic tone in which the fundamental and lower harmonics are absent.

VI. AIR SAC PRESSURES AND THE HÉRISSANT EFFECT

We earlier noted that a syrinx is exposed on all but its dorsal surface to the interclavicular air sac. This arrangement clearly provides space for syringeal movements and oscillation of syringeal membranes, but an even more intricate relationship exists. Hérissant[68] discovered that rupture of the interclavicular air sac drastically reduced the ability of a bird to vocalize. In a classic series of experiments many years later, Rüppell[54] attempted to obtain sounds from a Gull syrinx suspended in a glass chamber. He determined that a high pressure in the chamber was necessary for the induction of sound. These experiments led to the supposition that movement of the membranes into the lumen was at least in part due to an externally applied pressure. However, Rüppell's apparatus incorporated two flaws. First, the air supplies to the syrinx and to the chamber were independent, whereas they are contiguous in a bird (Figure 1). Thus, he could create conditions in which the static pressures on either side of the syringeal membranes were different, but a transmural pressure differential is possible in a bird only when flow induces a Bernoulli effect. Second, the syrinx in Rüppell's apparatus was essentially immobile. Gross[69] performed similar experiments using Chicken syringes and a chamber designed to replicate avian anatomy more closely. He also tested syringes set at different degrees of relaxation. His experiments determined that, for sound production, pressure in the chamber must at least equal that in the syrinx and that the required pressure

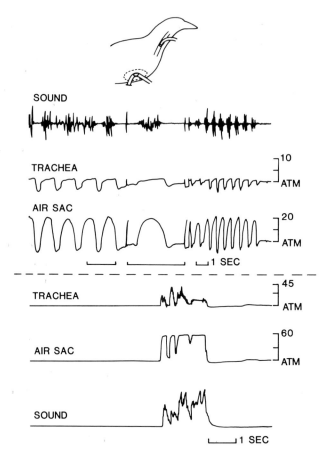

SOUND

TRACHEA

AIR SAC

TRACHEA

AIR SAC

SOUND

FIGURE 4.   Pressure in the air sacs and trachea during distress calls of a Starling (above) and crowing of a Rooster. Cartoon shows the placement of cannulae in the Starling, and the placement was comparable in the Chicken. Note that tracheal pressure during the distress call of the Starling scarcely exceeds atmospheric pressure (ATM), suggesting a tight closure. The pressure in the trachea of the Rooster more closely parallels both internal pressure and sound intensity. Pressure is measured in cmH_2O. (Based on References 70 and 71.)

increased as membrane tension rose. Higher chamber pressures required higher driving pressures in the bronchi for phonation. It follows that shortening the syrinx and relaxing the membranes reduced the required pressures in both bronchi and chamber. However, when the syrinx was fully collapsed, the required driving pressure suddenly increased 40-fold. Presumably at full contraction the infolding membranes press together and occlude the syringeal lumen. Then they must behave as pulse generators. Such a tight closure may be used by some Roosters for some calls that show little flow,[70] but the relatively high flow that is always present during crowing suggests that this call uses a less constricted configuration. It is well to remember, however, that the driving pressure head during crowing is extraordinarily high (Figure 4).[29,70]

Gaunt et al.[71] showed that when the interclavicular air sac of a Starling (*Sturnus vulgaris*) was opened, not only was the bird silenced, but flow through the syrinx virtually stopped. This and other evidence (Figure 4) led them to conclude that the songbird syrinx forms a tight valve during distress calls, and the air takes the path of least resistance through the cannula. However, this explanation does not work for Chickens, which remain silent even if all ostea leading into the interclavicular air sac are blocked.[10] In the absence of a counterbalancing external pressure, the syringeal membranes of a Chicken balloon outward during exhalation. These two situations provide a prime example of a common phenomenon in syringeal studies — similar effects may derive from quite different causes.

Just as the ''Hérissant effect'' may devolve from different causes in different species, so the effect itself is not uniform. Ducks in particular show different reactions depending on age and sex.[72,73] Lockner and Murrish[73] attribute the minimal effect in Drakes to the presence of a bulla peculiar to the syringes of many male anatids. The function of that bulla remains in question, but it tends to reduce rather than augment sound intensity and to insure that the vocal folds of a Drake's syrinx act as pulse generators.[11]

VII. MINIBREATHS, SOUND VALVES, AND THEIR INTERACTIONS

A. Prolonged Song

Many birds, especially songbirds, possess the ability to produce apparently uninterrupted sound for remarkably long periods of time; e.g., 27 sec for a Canary (*Serinus canaria*),[74] 41 sec for a Winter Wren (*Troglodytes troglodytes*),[75] and up to 117 sec for a Grasshopper Warbler (*Locustella naevia*).[76] A key word here is ''apparently'', because sonographic analysis of many songs reveals numerous interruptions that are sufficiently brief not to be perceived by human ears. Even so, some prolonged songs, e.g., that of the Grasshopper Warbler, are continuous, or the breaks are sufficiently brief to render their use for inhalation questionable. Further, the Winter Wren produces sound intensities of up to 90 dB at 1 m.[77] Using the formula of Lasiewsi and Calder[78] and weights provided by Brackenbury,[76] this author calculates the total respiratory volume of the Winter Wren as only 2.5 mℓ and that of the Grasshopper Warbler about 2.7 mℓ. Hence, some small birds are capable of truly prodigious performances.

An obvious explanation for such endurance is that the birds may vocalize during the entire respiratory cycle rather than just during exhalation. For example, Ring Doves (*Streptopelia risoria*)[48] often vocalize during the deep inhalations following calls. The occurrence of these apparently inadvertent sounds seems to increase with excitement and may actually serve a signal function. However, the only bird for which there is good evidence that inhalatory vocalization is a deliberate ploy is the Nightjar (*Caprimulgus europeaus*), which can vocalize continuously for up to 8 min. Frequency remains relatively constant throughout the song, but amplitude waxes and wanes with a periodicity equivalent to the respiratory frequency.[79]

Calder[74] proposed another mechanism to explain some of these improbable performances: a bird might extend its singing time by engaging in rapid, partial inhalations between notes or phrases. The ''minibreath'' hypothesis has enjoyed considerably popularity and has been adopted as at least a partial explanation of features of the songs of several species. Calder based his suggestions on data taken from a Canary that had been fitted with an impedance pneumograph. The data clearly showed rapid, shallow fluctuations of thoracic impedance synchronized with the notes of the bird's song, including the individual notes of a trill with a pulse rate of 25 Hz.

Unfortunately, Calder's procedure contained a serious, though not necessarily fatal, flaw. The output of an impedance pneumograph is not referenced to any external value, and the measured impedance can change with every change of the subject's bodily position, a fact that is quite evident in Calder's published oscillograms. In order for flow to reverse, even for an instant, the internal pressure of the bird must drop below ambient. But it is impossible to tell from Calder's data whether the impedance changes signify changes in thoracic volume sufficient to reverse flow, and in some cases the oscillograms strongly suggest that the changes are not sufficient.

B. Modulatory Effects

Although Calder's data do not demonstrate flow reversal, they distinctly implicate respiratory motions in the generation of sound modulations.[80] However, at least three other mechanisms are consistent with the data: (1) a dual-chambered system in which the inner (air sacs) and outer (pharynx) chambers expand and contract reciprocally; (2) a continuous input and unidirectional flow that is interrupted by an oscillating valve; and (3) a consistently high, but fluctuating driving pressure that produces a unidirectional, pulsatile flow.[70] The first of these seems improbable in birds, although it may occur in anurans.[34] An interrupted flow pattern commensurate with either of the latter two models has been recorded during trilling calls of the Evening Grosbeak (*Hesperophona vespertina*)[81] and the Starling,[71] and one or both of these mechanisms has since been implicated or demonstrated as the basis of amplitude modulation in a wide variety of calls.

An oscillating valve has been proposed as the mechanism of trilling in toads,[34] in which the arytenoid cartilages of the larynx are set into oscillation by the same airflow that drives the vocal folds. The opening and closing of the glottal opening alternately muffles sound or permits its free passage. As far as is known, the glottis of a bird is always open during phonation, but, according to the type of syrinx, either the lateral tympanic membranes or various structures associated with bronchial bars (e.g., lateral labia) may be appropriately positioned to perform a similar role.

A valve or interference mechanism in an extreme form has been demonstrated in the Grey Swiftlet, *Collocalia spodiopygia* (Figures 5 and 6). The echolocating cry of this bird is a double click. Suthers and Hector[82] provide simultaneous records of flow, pressure, and electromyograms of the syringeal muscles during calling. Pressure during a cry rises and falls smoothly and continuously, but flow ceases abruptly between the two clicks. EMG activity is strong in the sternotrachealis until the first click, then ceases as activity builds rapidly in the tracheolateralis. Suthers and Hector propose that contraction of the sternotrachealis relaxes the syrinx as pressure and flow build. This movement rotates the first bronchial cartilage into the lumen, forming a venturi-like slot that increases the Bernoulli effect opposite the medial tympanic membrane, which is thereby set into vibration, producing the first click. As the cartilage continues to rotate inward, it meets the medial tympanic membrane, blocking the lumen and stopping vibration. Now the activity of the tracheolateralis extends the syrinx and withdraws the bronchial cartilage. Flow is reestablished and a second click is produced. In this species, the phonatory pattern is a simple extension of the respiratory rhythm, and changes of syringeal configuration are of prime importance. The sequence of syringeal muscle contractions in Swiftlets exactly meets the expectations of classic models of syringeal action.

Suthers and Hector[82a] propose a slightly different mechanism for the production of echolocating clicks by the Oilbird (*Steatornis caripensis*). First, the anatomy of the vocal organs of an Oilbird is different in that they are entirely bronchial and include an intrinsic muscle. Differential action of that muscle (1) allows the system to act in a manner similar to the Swiftlet syrinx to produce double clicks, or (2) permits only the initial click by rapidly reopening the syrinx, or (3) holds the syrinx partially open, thereby permitting a continuous string of clicks. Oilbirds can also utter nonclicking squawks, which presumably require yet another setting of the syringeal configuration.

Pure versions of the third alternative, a fluctuating, driving pressure, are difficult to find. The rise and fall of activity in the abdominal muscles of a crowing Rooster more closely matches the divisions of sound than the activity in the syringeal muscles,[12] but those divisions are considerably coarser than the rapid modulations reported by Calder. Phillips and Youngren[83] showed pulsatile activity of the respiratory muscles during the fear-trill of a Chick. Here the pulse rate reaches 50 Hz, or twice that of a Canary's trill. We have repeated their experiments in conjunction with pressure measurements and determined that air sac pressures were always well above atmospheric.[43] The oscillations associated with individual notes

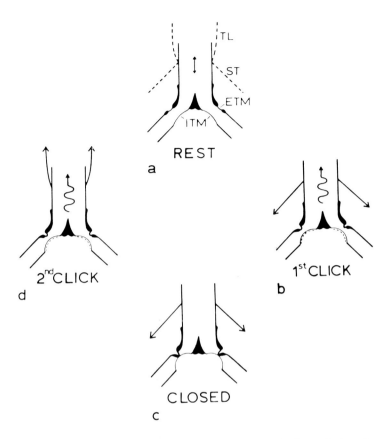

FIGURE 5.   Diagram showing the cycle of events responsible for production of a double click by *Collocalia*. Action of the tracheal muscles is indicated by arrows from tracheal wall. Airflow is indicated by arrow within trachea. Abbreviations: ETM, external (= lateral) tympanic membrane, ITM, internal (= medial) tympanic membrane; ST, sternotrachealis; TL, tracheolateralis. (From Suthers, R. and Hector, D. H., *J. Comp. Physiol.*, 148, 457, 1982. With permission.)

appear as ripples in the pressure curve. The pattern of activity in the syringeal muscles during this call is unknown.

Another possible example is the Skylark (*Alauda arvensis*), which sings while flying. Its song is divided into a series of phrases that are, in turn, subdivided into pulses. Neither the phrases nor the pulses correlate with the wing beat, but the intervals between phrases occur with a periodicity about that expected for ventilations.[84] Moreover, the length of the intervals is positively correlated with the length of the preceding phrase, which suggests a replenishing inhalation. The slowly pulsed phrases are distinct trills to the human ear. Brackenbury[85] has suggested that the pulses within the phrases represent ''high-frequency respiratory oscillations'' much like minibreaths, that presumably produce a series of air pulses like those of the Evening Grosbeak.

Brackenbury[76,80] provides two more cases that permit us to expand on this theme. The song of the Grasshopper Sparrow appears to combine elements of the preceding two cases. The song is a train of double clicks that often continues uninterrupted for periods of about 1 min. Brackenbury hypothesized that the two clicks represent a syringeal mechanism with the sternotrachealis and tracheolateralis acting much as in the Grey Swiftlet (Figure 6). The interclick interval is, thus, a period in which the syringeal lumen and flow are blocked. However, the oscine sternotrachealis is extremely small, especially in comparison to the

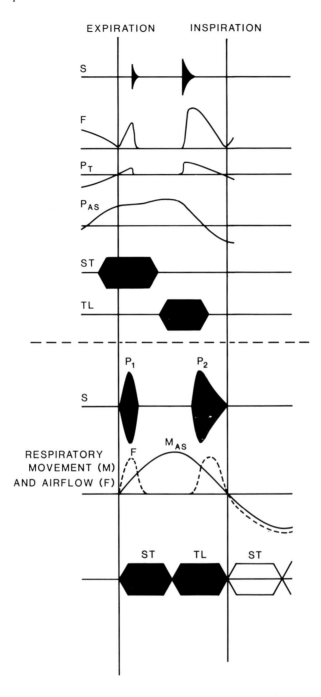

FIGURE 6.   A comparison of the models proposed for the production of double clicks by *Collocalia*[82] (top) and *Locustella*.[75] Both of the original drawings have been modified to emphasize similarities. Because the continued activity of the muscles during inhalation in Brackenbury's model seems questionable, those EMG pulses have not been "filled in". Abbreviations: F, flow; M_{AS}, respiratory compression of air sacs; P_{AS}, pressure in air sacs; P_T, pressure in trachea; ST, activity of sternotrachealis; TL, activity of tracheolateralis.

intrinsic muscles, and this author seriously doubts that it could function as Brackenbury suggested. Moreover, cutting the sternotrachealis will not prevent many birds, including songbirds, from uttering reasonably normal songs and calls.[29,86] It seems more likely that an Oscine would exploit the complexity of its syrinx by rotating the lateral labium (which is controlled by intrinsic muscles) in and out of the lumen against the vibrating medial tympanic membrane. Alternatively, the labium could be moved into the airstream and be itself driven into oscillation by airflow. Because of its mass, it would oscillate more slowly than the tympanic membrane. Thus, its action would induce a relatively slow modulation of a higher carrier frequency as proposed by Stein.[37] Brackenbury proposed that each double-click-plus-interclick interval represented a complete respiratory cycle. Because the interclick pause is so short, it seems unlikely to be a full inhalation. Hence, if this species can be induced to sing while instrumented, it would be a prime target to determine if minibreaths can function as Calder conceived.

More complicated yet is the song of the Sedge Warbler (*Acrocephalus schoenobaenus*), which also consists of trains of amplitude modulations (Figure 7). The trains are divided into phrases, each of which consists of a series of identical chirps, and each chirp contains a set of identical pulses. The temporal characteristics of each of these subdivisions are variable. When the modulations become very fast, the AM is incomplete, and the pulses may fuse to produce only ripples in the sound envelope. Brackenbury proposed that each train is produced during a single exhalation with the pauses between trains being inhalations. The chirps represent a second order of respiratory movement that divides the flow. The different phrases represent different frequencies of this secondary respiratory movement. He attributed the intrachirp pulses to activity of the syringeal muscles.

A major question is the nature of the syringeal activity. Brackenbury suggests that complete, or "true" pulses, with repetition rates of 25 to 90 Hz, are produced by alternating contractions of the extrinsic muscles, while the faster ripples (modal value of 320 Hz) are produced by intrinsic muscles, possibly operating at resonant frequencies. Again, this author doubts the proposed role of the extrinsic muscles and suspects that all syringeal changes are attributable to intrinsic musculature. As before, the lateral labium could be moved into the airstream by rotation of a bronchial bar. Close inspection of Brackenbury's Plates II and III shows that the respiratory and syringeal movements are not completely synchronized, and that the changes in pulse rate may themselves follow a cyclic pattern, as if the syringeal muscles were more-or-less rhythmically adjusting syringeal configuration. The lateral labium is continuous with a flexible, though rather heavy, membranous structure, the lateral tympanic membrane. Supposing the tension of the lateral tympanic membrane is adjustable by action of the intrinsic muscles, then the oscillatory properties of the attached labium could be adjusted. The slower, complete pulses could be produced by individual movements of the lateral labium into the lumen, and the faster, incomplete ripples by passive, flow-driven oscillations of the labium.

Although the foregoing examples are based solely on an analysis of the acoustics of the calls, the coo of the Ring Dove has been analyzed using both physiologic and electromyographic evidence.[48] The coo of the dove is composed of one or two introductory hoots followed by a prolonged portion (Figure 7). The prolonged portion begins with a series of regular pulses that gradually increase in both amplitude and duration, and thus sounds distinctly warbled. Eventually the sound becomes relatively continuous, or at least fluctuates irregularly. Oscillograms of both the pulsed and continuous portions show the presence of a second, less complete AM that divides the sound envelope into a series of ellipsoids. The continuous portion is rich in timbre although it contains no overtones. The beginning and end of the continuous portion may also contain a series of very brief, sharp pulses. These can be shown to be beats resulting from the presence of two, slightly different frequencies. Presumably one frequency is produced by each side of the syrinx; i.e., this seeming modulation is actually a product of the two-voice phenomenon and not a true modulation.

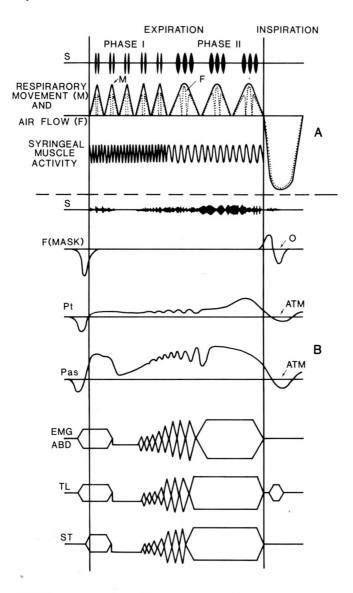

FIGURE 7. A comparison of the models proposed for sound production in *Acrocephalus*[76] (top) and *Streptopelia*.[48] See text for discussion. Abbreviations: ABD, activity in abdominal compressor muslces; other abbreviations as in Figure 6.

The major pulses during the warbled portion of the call are generated by action of the ventilatory musculature. Each pulse is associated with a burst of EMG activity in the abdominal compressor muscles and a distinct oscillation of pressure in the air sac. In some individuals, this basic pattern may be augmented by pulsatile activity of the syringeal muscles.

The ellipsoidal oscillations are spread throughout the call with no reference to changes in the activity pattern of any muscle. If the sound originates in the vicinity of the medial membranes, then oscillations of the more cranial lateral membranes could alter the diameter of the trachea, alternately permitting or impeding the free passage of sound in a manner similar to that supposed for bronchial bars of the Grey Swiftlet or the lateral labia of the Sedge Warbler. In Doves, the maximum impedance is rarely complete. As this modulatory pattern is not associated with regular muscular activity, we can assume that the vibrations of the lateral membranes are also driven by the airflow.

Not all AM is imparted by ventilatory events. In the Parrot *Myiopsitta monachus,* the driving pressure is relatively constant, but the intrinsic syringeal muscles show contractions that match the sound pulses. Here modulations can be attributed primarily to changes in syringeal configuration,[9] changes that include the imposition of a pair of unusual syringeal flaps into the airstream.[87] We presume that these flaps function as an oscillating valve much in the manner proposed for the Grey Swiftlet, Sedge Warbler, and Ring Dove. Indeed, the presence of a secondary syringeal oscillator that divides more-or-less continuous sounds in a series of pulses seems to be very common.[43] These oscillators may be either passively driven by airflow or actively moved by muscular action.

It is curious that the majority of modulatory patterns that have thus far been analyzed involved AM, despite the fact that a mechanism for FM seems so obvious. Suthers and Hector[82] describe an FM pattern in surgically altered *Collocalia* that could be accounted for by passive responses of the oscillating membranes to changes in the driving pressure and/ or flow.[43] Such "passive" processes must be responsible for those modulations of both frequency and amplitude seen in the calls of birds in which the syringeal muscles have been denervated.[11] The only FM pattern so far linked to the action of syringeal muscles is a shift in pitch during a disyllabic call of the Peach-Faced Lovebird, *Agapornis roseicollis.*[9]

VIII. ENERGETICS

Phonation is a behavioral technique whereby an animal can extend its physical presence. Clearly it takes far less energy for a bird to defend a given volume of space by filling it with song than by patrolling its periphery. Unfortunately, little information exists about the actual cost of phonation to a bird. Despite considerable effort in our laboratory, we have been unable to detect any change in the rate of the oxygen consumption of a Canary during singing,[88] suggesting that the effort is scarcely greater than "background". However, the technical problems associated with that study are such that further experimentation would be prudent before drawing firm conclusions.

A Rooster converts something less than 2% of the fluid energy generated by compression of its air sacs into energy. Such an ineffective performance may derive from the high threshold airflow velocity necessary to prevent inadvertent triggering of membrane oscillation, especially during panting or periods of exercise.[29,89,90] Certainly one of the functions of the extrinsic syringeal musculature is to maintain the patency of the airway during periods of high flow.[10,15,19] Given the lethal possibilities of an obstructed airway, redundant safety factors are to be expected. That explanation, however, does not explain why the crow of a Rooster requires driving pressures almost double those of birds of comparable size uttering sounds of comparable intensity (Tables 1 and 2).

As mentioned in Section II.C, vocal plasticity depends on the presence of intrinsic musculature, but the complexity of that musculature bears no simple relationship to vocal virtuosity. Evidently complex syringeal musculature arose under a selective regime for some other capability. Although that capability might be an as yet undetected ventilatory function, some other aspect of vocal physiology seems a more parsimonious hypothesis. Intrinsic musculature may promote vocalization that is more effective in terms of the sound produced as a function of either air exhaled[59,70,71] or energy consumed.[29,89,90] Roosters use more than 90% of their ventilatory capacity during a single challenge call,[29,89] whereas Starlings use less than 20% during loud distress calling.[71] The ability of songbirds to sing for prolonged periods has already been discussed (Section VII.A).

Because the driving force for phonation ultimately derives from contraction of the abdominal muscles, we might expect that the power of the radiated sound would increase with

Table 1
AIR SAC PRESSURES DURING CALLS OF
SEVERAL SPECIES

Species	Call	Air sac pressure (cmH$_2$O)
Sturnus vulgaris[71] Starling	Distress	18—30
Cyanocitta cristata Blue Jay	Bugle Jay	19.2 ± 1.3 25—>30
Myiopsitta monachus Monk Parakeet	Squawk	35.4 ± 1.7
Streptopelia risoria[48] Ring Dove	Whinny Coo	15—36 15—38
Anas platyrhynchos Mallard—young[73] —adult[70,73]	Peep Rab-Rab	26 ± 1.5 10 ± 1.5; 5—10
Anthropoides virgo[50] Demoiselle Crane	Alarm	36.6 ± 2.2
Gallus gallus[29,70] Domestic Chicken	Cluck Crow	5—25 50—60
Balaerica pavonina[50] Western Crowned Crane	Alarm	24.9 ± 3.3
Anser anser[29] Domestic Goose	Honk	20—30
Grus canadenis[50] Sandhill Crane	Alarm	20.3 ± 1.1
Grus vipio[50] White-Naped Crane	Alarm	30.0 ± 2.0
Grus rubicunda[50] Brolga	Alarm	17.7 ± 1.4

Note: When possible, data are presented as a mean ± 1 SE; otherwise a range is provided. Note that a Rooster's crows are always loud, whereas the calls of other birds may be of variable intensities and therefore use a greater range of driving pressures. Data from the Blue Jay and Monk Parakeet are from the author's files. Other data are from the literature as indicated.

increasing size. Certainly size is an influencing factor (Table 2). The sound intensity of Crane calls varies both with size and with the degree of tracheal coiling. In Oscines, larger birds generally produce louder calls, but small songbirds often appear to be even less effective than expected.[77] Brackenbury organized his data in order of decreasing sound intensity. When the same data are reordered by decreasing body weight, and if additional data are included, the relationship between size and sound output, although generally present, is less convincing. This is an area in which additional data could be easily obtained and would be of considerable interest.

To some extent, the amount of sound radiated may depend on the impedance match between the generating system and the surrounding medium. When crowing, a Rooster lowers its hyoid apparatus and greatly expands its pharynx, converting the pharyngobuccal chamber into a form that could help match impedance between the vocal tract and the environment, much in the manner of the bell of a brass instrument or a megaphone.[35,91] Roosters and other large birds that can generate extremely high flow rates may be able to

Table 2
SOUND INTENSITIES OF AVIAN VOCALIZATIONS
COMPARED WITH BODY WEIGHT

Species	Weight (g)	Sound intensity		
		dB	mW	mW/Kg
Homo sapiens	72,600	103	120	1.7
Author				
Grus antigone (5)	10,800	116	2390	221
Sarus Crane				
Bugaranus leucogeranus (1)	7,000	106	239	34
Siberian Crane				
Grus rubincunda (6)	6,200	118	3790	640
Brolga				
Grus canadensis (4)	4,500	108	379	84
Sandhill Crane				
Balaerica pavonina (0)	4,400	110	601	137
Western Crowned Crane				
*Gallus gallus**	3,500	105	190	54
Domestic Chicken				
Cyanoleuca patagonia	240	101	76	317
Patagonian Parrot				
Streptopelia risoria	155	80	6	3.9
Ring Dove				
Myiopsitta monachus	130	95	19	146
Monk Parakeet				
*Turdus merula**	96	87	3	30
European Blackbird				
*Turdus philomelos**	69	100	60	870
Song Thrush				
*Emberiza citrinella**	28	85	2	70
Yellowhammer				
*Fringilla coelebs**	22	86	3	135
Chaffinch				
*Erithacus rubecula**	20	90	6	300
Robin				
*Emberiza schoeniclus**	20	78	0.4	20
Reed Bunting				
Serinus canaria	19	79	0.5	26
Canary				
*Acanthis cannabina**	19	75	0.2	10
Linnet				
*Sylvia atricappilla**	18	88	4	220
Blackcap				
*Sylvia communis**	15	74	0.15	10
Whitethroat				
*Locustella naevia**	12	85	2	165
Grasshopper Warbler				
*Sylvia curruca**	12	80	0.6	50
Lesser Whitethroat				
*Acrocephalus schoenobaenus**	11	80	0.6	55
Sedge Warbler				

Table 2 (continued)
SOUND INTENSITIES OF AVIAN VOCALIZATIONS
COMPARED WITH BODY WEIGHT

Species	Weight (g)	Sound intensity		
		dB	mW	mW/Kg
*Troglodytes troglodytes** Wren	10	90	6	600
*Phylloscopus collybitus** Chiffchaff	9	80	0.6	65
*Parus ater** Coal Tit	9	78	0.4	45
*Phylloscopus trachilus** Willow Warbler	8	77	0.3	40
*Regulus regulus** Goldcrest	6	75	0.2	35

Note: All dB measures have been adjusted to a distance of 1 m from source. A human shout has been included for comparison. The dB readings were converted to milliwatts by the method of Brackenbury.[29] Asterisk data are from Brackenbury,[77] crane data are taken from Gaunt et al.[50] Other data are from the author's files.

achieve "convective coupling", in which the sound waves in the vocal tract are magnified by the velocity of the conducting airstream.[39,90]

Several species of birds, most of which have low, booming calls, possess diverticula of the trachea or esophagus that are inflated during vocalization. The role(s) of these vocal sacs has (have) not been experimentally determined. In Doves, the vocal sac does not determine the pitch of the call but does seem to affect sound intensity.[48] It is possible that vocal sacs serve to increase the surface area from which a sound is radiated, thereby functioning in a manner analogous to the sound board of a string instrument. Conversely, it is possible that some sound sacs and the syringeal bullae of male anatids may serve as side-branch mufflers to damp certain frequencies.[11,35] The large coiled trachea in some birds that are noted for their ability to utter extremely loud calls may also enhance sound radiation. In some species, the enlarged trachea lies immediately beneath the skin,[92] where it may radiate directly to the air; in others it is imbedded in the sternum, which in turn presses against the air sacs, much like the sounding board of a violin or guitar.[50]

IX. SUMMARY

Because the vocal systems of tetrapods are all derivatives of the ventilatory system, they are bound to share certain attributes. Hence, it is hardly surprising that the gross intensities of vocalizations in all tetrapods are ultimately determined by activity of the respiratory musculature. In birds, however, the integration of ventilatory structures and functions into the vocal process is far more extensive. Compression of the ventilatory system not only provides the driving pressure head but is also partially responsible for reshaping the syrinx into a vocalizing configuration. Emerging from many studies is a theme of interlocking ventilatory and syringeal movements that can produce intricate patterns of AM, even in the absence of complex syringeal musculature or two voices. There is reason to suspect that at least some FM may derive from similar interactions.

Although we can now offer some generalizations about the mechanics of some vocal phenomena, generalizing about the distribution of those mechanisms remains dangerous.

Even Parrots in the same subfamily,[9] or Sandpipers in the same genus,[43,93] may differ in syringeal structure and/or may use those structures in different ways. Roosters (a rooster?) may produce similar sounds by using different techniques.[12]

If this review is an accurate view of current knowledge, then the throughtful reader will quickly agree with Brackenbury[90] that, "Many of the ideas about the function of the passerine syrinx are based on informed guesswork". This author, however, would not limit that assessment to passerines.

Much remains to be learned. In particular, we are woefully ignorant of the nature of syringeal movements, especially the configurations and modes of vibration of syringeal membranes, in *any* intact bird. The technical problems involved in acquiring such data are formidable, but the problem might be approachable by a combination of EBS and fiber-optic techniques. We have no information on the role(s), if any, of resonances, of the air sacs and skeleton, especially the sternum. At the onset of the breeding season, many birds devote a significant portion of their time to vocal performances, yet virtually nothing is known of the energetic costs of that activity. Students of communication who are willing and able to blend physiology and behavior will find that the study of avian phonation provides questions and opportunities in abundance.

ACKNOWLEDGMENTS

Only sheer arrogance would allow me to pretend that the themes and interpretations of this review are entirely my own. Time and again, I have found that notions I considered original had been directly stated or strongly implied by others, although sometimes in terms that I had not appreciated until my own thinking had matured. If that new "appreciation" has led me to infer meanings that were not implied, I apologize. I have benefitted greatly from discussions and correspondence with many colleagues and students, and often find it difficult to determine where my interpretations begin and theirs end, or who was originally responsible for what. Hence, it seems inappropriate to single out a few from the many for special thanks. However, little that I have accomplished would have been possible without the reorientation of my approach to research effected under the guidance of Carl Gans, and the help, encouragement, and occasional goading of my wife Sandra L. L. Gaunt.

David Dennis drew Figure 2 and helped prepare the other illustrations for this paper. Our work on Cranes, some of which is reported here, and the production of this review were aided by grants from the National Science Foundation (PCM-8302203) and the National Geographic Society (2626-83).

REFERENCES

1. **Vince, M. A.**, Embryonic communication, in *Bird Vocalization,* Hinde, R. A., Ed., Cambridge University Press, London, 1969, chap. 11.
2. **Beddard, F. E.**, *The Structure and Classification of Birds,* Longman, Green & Co., New York, 1898.
3. **Ames, P. L.**, The morphology of the syrinx in birds, *Peabody Mus. Nat. Hist. Yale Univ. Bull.*, 37, 1, 1971.
4. **Warner, R. W.**, The Anatomy of the Avian Syrinx, Ph.D. thesis, University of London, 1969. (Microfilm available for loan from Center for Research Libraries, Chicago, Ill.)
5. **Warner, R. W.**, The structural basis of the organ of voice in the genera *Anas* and *Aythya* (Aves), *J. Zool.*, 164, 197, 1971.
6. **Warner, R. W.**, The syrinx in the family Columbidae, *J. Zool.*, 166, 385, 1972.
7. **Warner, R. W.**, The anatomy of the syrinx in passerine birds, *J. Zool.*, 168, 381, 1972.
8. **Nottebohm, F.**, Phonation in the orange-winged Amazon parrot, *Amazona amazonia, J. Comp. Physiol.*, 108, 157, 1976.

9. **Gaunt, A. S. and Gaunt, S. L. L.,** Electromyographic studies of the syrinx in parrots (Aves, Psittacidae), *Zoomorphology,* 105, 1, 1985.
10. **Youngren, O. M., Peek, F. W., and Phillips, R. E.,** Repetitive vocalizations evoked by local electrical stimulation of avian brains. III. Evoked activity in the tracheal muscles of the Chicken (*Gallus gallus*), *Brain Behav. Evol.,* 9, 393, 1974.
11. **Lockner, F. R. and Youngren, O. M.,** Functional syringeal anatomy of the Mallard. I. *In situ* electromyograms during ESB elicited calling, *Auk,* 93, 324, 1976.
12. **Gaunt, A. S. and Gaunt, S. L. L.,** Mechanics of the syrinx in *Gallus gallus.* II. Electromyographic studies of *ad libitum* vocalizations, *J. Morphol.,* 152, 1, 1977.
13. **Gaunt, A. S.,** An hypothesis concerning the relationship of syringeal structure to vocal abilities, *Auk,* 100, 853, 1983.
14. **Mongue, K. R. and Nottebohm, F.,** Relation of medullary motor nuclei to nerves supplying the vocal-tract in the Budgerigar (*Melopsittacus undulatus*), *J. Comp. Physiol.,* 204, 384, 1982.
15. **Nottebohm, F.,** Neural lateralization of vocal control in a passerine bird. I. Song, *J. Exp. Zool.,* 177, 299, 1971.
16. **Nottebohm, F.,** Neural lateralization of vocal control in a passerine bird. II. Subsong, calls, and a theory of vocal learning, *J. Exp. Zool.,* 179, 35, 1972.
17. **Lemon, R. E.,** Nervous control of the syrinx in White-throated Sparrows (*Zonotrichia albicollis*), *J. Zool.,* 171, 131, 1973.
18. **Nottebohm, F. and Nottebohm, M. E.,** Left hypoglossal dominance in the control of Canary and White-crowned Sparrow song, *J. Comp. Physiol.,* 108, 171, 1976.
19. **Seller, T. J.,** Unilateral nervous control of the syrinx in Java Sparrows (*Padda oryzivora*), *J. Comp. Physiol.,* 129, 281, 1979.
20. **Peek, F. W.,** An experimental study of the territorial function of vocal and visual display in the male Redwinged Blackbird (*Agelaius phoenicus*), *Anim. Behav.,* 20, 112, 1972.
21. **Smith, D. G.,** An experimental analysis of the function of Redwinged Blackbird song, *Behaviour,* 56, 136, 1976.
22. **Phillips, R. E., Youngren, O. M., and Peek, F. W.,** Repetitive vocalizations evoked by local electrical brain stimulation of avian brains. I. Awake Chickens *(Gallus gallus), Anim. Behav.,* 20, 689, 1972.
23. **Peek, F. W. and Phillips, R. E.,** Repetitive vocalizations evoked by local electrical stimulation of avian brains. II. Anesthetized Chickens *(Gallus gallus), Brain Behav. Evol.,* 4, 417, 1971.
24. **Peek, F. W., Youngren, O. M., and Phillips, R. E.,** Repetitive vocalizations evoked by local electrical stimulation of avian brains. IV. Evoked and spontaneous activity in expiratory and inspiratory nerves and muscles of the Chicken *(Gallus gallus), Brain Behav. Evol.,* 12, 1, 1975.
25. **Maley, M. J.,** Electrical stimulation of agonistic behaviour in the Mallard, *Behaviour,* 34, 138, 1969.
26. **Potash, L. M.,** Neuroanatomical regions relevant to production and analysis of vocalization within the avian *torus semicircularis, Experientia,* 26, 1104, 1970.
27. **Brown, J. L.,** An exploratory study of vocalization areas in the brain of the Redwinged Blackbird *(Agealius phoenicius), Behaviour,* 39, 91, 1971.
28. **Brown, J. L.,** Behavior elicited by electrical stimulation of the brain of Steller's Jay, *Condor,* 75, 1, 1973.
29. **Brackenbury, J. H.,** Respiratory mechanics of sound production in chickens and geese, *J. Exp. Biol.,* 72, 229, 1978.
30. **Richards, S. A.,** Brain stem control of polypnoea in the Chicken and Pigeon, *Respir. Physiol.,* 11, 315, 1971.
31. **Arnold, A. P.,** Neural control of passerine song, in *Acoustic Communication in Birds,* Vol. 1, Kroodsma, D. E. and Miller, E. H., Eds., Academic Press, New York, 1982, chap. 3.
32. **Nottebohm, F.,** Birdsong as a model in which to study brain processes related to learning, *Condor,* 86, 227, 1984.
33. **Lieberman, P.,** *On the Origin of Language: An Introduction to the Evolution of Human Speech,* Macmillan, New York, 1975, chap. 5 to 7.
34. **Martin, W. M. and Gans, C.,** Muscular control of the vocal tract during release signalling in the toad *Bufo valliceps, J. Morphol.,* 137, 1, 1972.
35. **Rossing, T. D.,** *The Science of Sound,* Addison-Wesley, Reading, Mass., 1982, chap. 4, 11 through 13, and 15.
36. **Greenewalt, C. H.,** *Bird Song: Acoustics and Physiology,* Smithsonian Institute, Washington, D.C., 1968.
37. **Stein, R. C.,** Modulation in bird sounds, *Auk,* 85, 229, 1968.
38. **Chamberlain, D. R., Gross, W. B., Cornwell, G. W., and Mosby, H. S.,** Syringeal anatomy in the Common Crow, *Auk,* 85, 244, 1968.
39. **Brackenbury, J.,** Aeroacoustics of the vocal organ of birds, *J. Theor. Biol.,* 81, 341, 1979.
40. **Durrwang, R.,** Funktionelle Biologie, Anatomie und Physiologie der Vogelstimme, Ph.D. thesis, University of Basel, Basel, Switzerland, 1974.

41. **Klatt, D. H. and Stefanski, R. A.,** How does a mynah bird imitate human speech?, *J. Acoust. Soc. Am.,* 55, 822, 1974.
42. **Casey, R. M. and Gaunt, A. S.,** Theoretical models of the avian syrinx, *J. Theor. Biol.,* 116, 62, 1985.
43. **Gaunt, A. S. and Gaunt, S. L. L.,** Syringeal structure and avian phonation, in *Current Ornithology,* Vol. 2, Johnston, R. F., Ed., Plenum Press, New York, 1985, chap. 7.
44. **Paulsen, K.,** *Das Prinzip der Stimmbildung in der Wirbeltierreihe und beim Menschen,* Akad. Verlag, Frankfurt-am-Main, Germany 1967, chap. 9.
45. **Miskimen, M.,** Sound production in passerine birds, *Auk,* 68, 493, 1951.
46. **Gross, W. B.,** Devoicing the Chicken, *Poult. Sci.,* 43, 1143, 1964.
47. **Gross, W. B.,** An operation for reducing vocal intensity in the Peafowl, *Avian Dis.,* 23, 1031, 1979.
48. **Gaunt, A. S., Gaunt, S. L. L., and Casey, R. M.,** Syringeal mechanics reassessed: evidence from *Streptopelia, Auk,* 99, 474, 1982.
49. **van den Berg, Jw.,** Sound production in isolated human larynges, *Ann. N.Y. Acad. Sci.,* 155, 18, 1968.
50. **Gaunt, A. S., Gaunt, S. L. L., Prange, H. D., and Wasser, J.,** The effects of tracheal coiling on the vocalization of cranes (Aves; Gruidae), submitted.
51. **Abs, M.,** Zur Bioakustik der Stimmbruchs bei Vogeln, *Jahrb. Abt. Allg. Zool. Physiol.,* 84, 289, 1980.
52. **Hersh, G. L.,** Bird Voices and Resonant Tuning in Helium-Air Mixtures, Ph.D. thesis, University of California, Berkeley, 1967 (available from University Microfilms, Ann Arbor, Mich.).
53. **Myers, J. A.,** Studies on the syrinx of *Gallus domesticus, J. Morphol.,* 29, 165, 1917.
54. **Rüppell, W.,** Physiologie und Akustik der Vogelstimme, *J. Ornithol.,* 81, 433, 1933.
55. **Sutherland, C. A. and McChesney, D. S.,** Sound production in two species of geese, *Living Bird,* 4, 99, 1965.
56. **Würdinger, I.,** Erzeugung, Ontogenie und Funktion der Lautauserung bei den Ganseärten *(Anser indicus, A. caerulescens, A. albifrons* und *Branta canadensis), Z. Tierpsychol.,* 27, 257, 1970.
57. **Harris, C. L., Gross, W. B., and Robeson, A.,** Vocal acoustics of the Chicken, *Poult. Sci.,* 47, 107, 1968.
57a. **Roberts, L. H.,** Comparative Study of Sound Production in Small Mammals with Special Reference to Ultrasound, Ph.D. thesis, University of London, 1973.
57b. **Nowicki, S.,** Vocal tract resonances in oscine bird sound production: evidence from bird songs in a helium atmosphere, *Nature,* 325, 53, 1987.
58. **Hinsch, K.,** Akustik Gegansanalysis beim Fitis *(Phylloscopus trochilus)* zur Untersuchung der Rolle der Luftrohre bei der Stimmerzeugung der Singvogel, *J. Ornithol.,* 113, 315, 1972.
59. **Gaunt, A. S. and Wells, M. K.,** Models of syringeal mechanisms, *Am. Zool.,* 13, 1227, 1973.
60. **Chanaud, R. S.,** Aerodynamic whistles, *Sci. Am.,* 222(1), 40, 1970.
61. **Beebe, [C.] W.,** The Variegated Tinamou, *Crypturus variagatus variagatus* (Gmelin), *Zoologica,* 6, 195, 1925.
62. **Wilson, T. A., Beavers, G. S., DeCoster, M. A., Holger, D. K., and Regenfuss, M. D.,** Experiments on the fluid mechanics of whistling, *J. Acoust. Soc. Am.,* 50, 366, 1971.
63. **Potter, R. K., Kopp, G. A., and Green, H. C.,** *Visible Speech,* D Van Nostrand, Princeton, N.J., 1947, 411.
64. **Borror, D. J. and Reese, C. R.,** Vocal gymnastics in Wood Thrush songs, *Ohio J. Sci.,* 56, 177, 1956.
65. **Thorpe, W. H.,** *Bird Song,* Cambridge University Press, London, 1961, 112.
66. **Miller, D. B.,** Two-voice phenomenon in birds: further evidence, *Auk,* 94, 567, 1977.
67. **Gaunt, A. S.,** On sonograms, harmonics, and assumptions, *Condor,* 85, 259, 1983.
67a. **Nowicki, S. and Capranica, R. R.,** Bilateral syringeal interaction in vocal production of an oscine bird sound, *Science,* 231, 1297, 1986.
68. **Hérissant, [F.-D.],** Recherches sur les organes de voix des quadrupédes et de celle des oiseaux, *Acad. R. Sci. Mem. Paris,* 279, 1753.
69. **Gross, W. B.,** Voice production by the Chicken, *Poult. Sci.,* 43, 1143, 1964.
70. **Gaunt, A. S., Gaunt, S. L. L., and Hector, D. H.,** Mechanics of the syrinx in *Gallus gallus.* I. A comparison of pressure events in Chickens to those in Oscines, *Condor,* 78, 208, 1976.
71. **Gaunt, A. S., Stein, R. C., and Gaunt, S. L. L.,** Pressure and air flow during distress calls of the Starling, *Sturnus vulgaris* (Aves: Passeriformes), *J. Exp. Zool.,* 183, 241, 1973.
72. **Gottlieb, G. and Vandenbergh, J. G.,** Ontogeny of vocalization in Mallard Duck embryos, *J. Exp. Zool.,* 168, 307, 1968.
73. **Lockner, F. R. and Murrish, D. E.,** Interclavicular air sac pressures and vocalization in Mallard Ducks *Anas platyrhynchos, Comp. Biochem. Physiol.,* 52, 183, 1975.
74. **Calder, W. A.,** Respiration during singing in the Canary *(Serinus canaria), Comp. Biochem. Physiol.,* 32, 251, 1970.
75. **Clark, R. B.,** Some statistical information about wren song, *Br. Birds,* 42, 337, 1949.

76. **Brackenbury, J. H.,** A comparison of the origin and temporal arrangement of pulsed sounds in the songs of the Grasshopper and Sedge Warblers, *Locustella naevia* and *Acrocephalus schoenobaenus, J. Zool.,* 184, 187, 1978.

77. **Brackenbury, J. H.,** Power capabilities of the avian sound-producing system, *J. Exp. Biol.,* 78, 163, 1979.

78. **Lasiewski, R. C. and Calder, W. A., Jr.,** A preliminary allometric analysis of respiratory variables in resting birds, *Respir. Physiol.,* 11, 152, 1971.

79. **Hunter, M. L., Jr.,** Vocalization during inhalation in a nightjar, *Condor,* 82, 101, 1980.

80. **Brackenbury, J.,** Respiration and production of sounds by birds, *Biol. Rev.,* 55, 363, 1980.

81. **Berger, M. and Hart, J. S.,** Ein Beitrag zum Zusammenhang zwischen Stimme und Atmung bei Vogeln, *J. Ornithol.,* 109, 421, 1968.

82. **Suthers, R. A. and Hector, D. H.,** Mechanism of the production of echolocating clicks by the Grey Swiftlet, *Collocalia spodiopygia, J. Comp. Physiol.,* 148A, 457, 1982.

82a. **Suthers, R. A. and Hector, D. H.,** The physiology of vocalization by the echolocating oilbird, *Steatornis caripensis, J. Comp. Physiol.,* 156A, 243, 1985.

83. **Phillips, R. E. and Youngren, O. M.,** Effects of the denervation of the tracheosyringeal muscles on frequency control in vocalizations of chicks, *Auk,* 98, 299, 1981.

84. **Csicsaky, M.,** Über den Gesang der Feldlerche *(Alauda arvensis)* und sein Beziehung zur Atmung, *J. Ornithol.,* 119, 249, 1978.

85. **Brackenbury, J. H.,** A possible relationship between respiratory movements, syringeal movements and production of song by Skylarks *Alauda arvensis, Ibis,* 120, 526, 1978.

86. **Smith, D. G.,** The role of the sternograchealis muscles in bird song production, *Auk,* 94, 152, 1977.

87. **Gaunt, S. L. L. and Gaunt, A. S.,** Syringeal Configuration in Parrots, poster paper at 101st Stated Meet., American Ornithologists' Union, September 26 to 30, New York, 1983.

88. **Cammilleri, T. J. and Gaunt, A. S.,** unpublished data.

89. **Brackenbury, J. H.,** Physiological energetics of cock-crow, *Nature (London),* 270, 433, 1977.

90. **Brackenbury, J. H.,** The structural basis of voice production and its relationship to sound characteristics, in *Acoustic Communication in Birds,* Vol. 1, Kroodsma, D. E. and Miller, E. H., Eds., Academic Press, New York, NY, 1982, chap. 2

91. **White, S. S.,** Movement of the larynx during crowing in the domestic cock, *J. Anat.,* 103, 390, 1968.

92. **Clench, M. H.,** Tracheal elongation in birds of paradise, *Condor,* 80, 423, 1978.

93. **Miller, E. H.,** The structure of aerial displays in three species of Calidridinae (Scolopacidae), *Auk,* 100, 440, 1983.

Section II: Physiology

Chapter 4

GAS EXCHANGE AND TRANSPORT

Peter Scheid and Johannes Piiper

TABLE OF CONTENTS

I. INTRODUCTION

The basic principles of anatomy and physiology of the respiratory system have been primarily developed for mammals, for which they are well known in essence. Lungs of birds are certainly to be considered as homologous to lungs of mammals, and both are phylogenetically derived from those of their reptilian ancestors. However, there exist fundamental differences in anatomical design, in respiratory gas flow pattern, and in gas exchange function between avian and mammalian lungs.

In mammals the bronchial tree is an extensively branching tube system, typically of dichotomous arrangement. The distal generations (respiratory bronchioles and alveolar ducts) bear alveoli which are surrounded by a network of pulmonary capillaries. In this system, the airflow direction obviously has to be inward in inspiration and outward during expiration. In bird lungs, however, alternative pathways for gas flow exist anatomically. Indeed, as will be shown, in the avian respiratory tract the flow events during expiration are by no means mere reversals of those during inspiration.

When blood perfuses the mammalian lung, it is brought into intimate contact with the alveolar gas space, and an almost perfect equilibrium is attained for the respiratory gases, O_2 and CO_2, between end-capillary blood and alveolar air (cf. Reference 1). As a result, partial pressures for O_2 and CO_2 in arterial blood, Pa_{O_2} and Pa_{CO_2}, are nearly the same as those in end-expired gas, PE'_{O_2} and PE'_{CO_2}. Only with pathological degrees of heterogeneity, venous admixture, or diffusion impairment will there be a significant "gap" between the ranges in gas and blood partial pressures, i.e., $Pa_{O_2} < PE'_{O_2}$, $Pa_{CO_2} > PE'_{CO_2}$.

In birds, it is often observed that Pa_{O_2} exceeds PE'_{O_2} and that Pa_{CO_2} is smaller than PE'_{CO_2}.[2-4] Thus, the gas and blood partial pressure ranges for both gases show an "overlap", particularly during hypercapnic hypoxia.

The difference between mammals and birds in the relative position of gas and blood partial pressure ranges suggests a qualitative difference in the type of gas exchange organ between the mammalian lung, in which the overlap does not occur under normal conditions (cf. References 1 and 5) and in the avian lung, in which the overlap is a typical observation.

II. GAS TRANSPORT IN THE RESPIRATORY SYSTEM

A. Anatomy of the Respiratory System

The anatomy of the respiratory tract has been treated in a number of recent articles and reviews.[6-12] The respiratory airways (Figure 1) comprise (1) the bronchial system (trachea, primary or main bronchi, and secondary bronchi); (2) the lung (parabronchi and air capillaries), which serves gas exchange; and (3) the air sacs, which allow the volume changes required for tidal ventilation without significant gas exchange across their walls.[13] Unlike the mammalian lung, the structural elements subserving ventilation and gas exchange are thus separated.

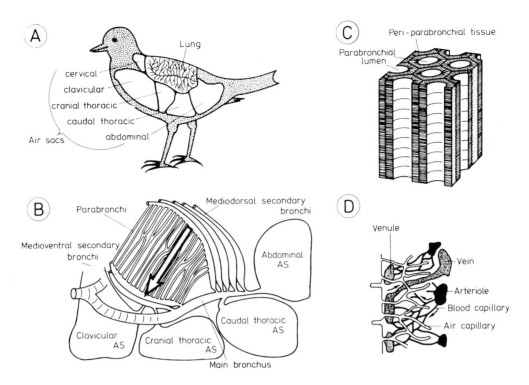

FIGURE 1. Scheme of respiratory system in birds. It comprises the lung and a number of air sacs (A and B). The lung is composed of long narrow tubes, parabronchi (A and C), through which gas flows in the same direction during both inspiration and expiration: from mediodorsal (dorsobronchi) to medioventral secondary bronchi (ventrobronchi; arrow in B). The periparabronchial tissue, a dense network of air capillaries and blood capillaries (D), constitutes the site for respiratory gas exchange. (Modified from Scheid.[27])

1. The Bronchial System

The trachea divides in the lower neck into the right and left main bronchi. After entering the lung, each main bronchus gives off a series of secondary bronchi, the medioventral secondary bronchi (referred to here as ventrobronchi), which occupy with extensive ramification the ventral surface of the lung. Between the ventrobronchi and the second set of secondary bronchi, the mediodorsal secondary bronchi (referred to here as dorsobronchi), there is only a short stretch of the main bronchus without openings to the secondary bronchi. The dorsobronchi and their branches form the dorsolateral surface of the lung. Additionally, there are lateroventral and laterodorsal secondary bronchi. The second lateroventral bronchus (laterobronchus) generally provides the direct connection to the caudal thoracic air sac (see below).

2. The Lungs

The two main sets of secondary bronchi, medioventral (ventrobronchi) and mediodorsal (dorsobronchi), are connected by the intrapulmonary airways, the tertiary bronchi or parabronchi, which are long, narrow tubes, displaying only a mild degree of anastomosing, around their origins from secondary bronchi and around the middle of their length (Figure 1). Parabronchi extend across the lungs, are thus about one to several cm in length, and their lumen is about 1 mm wide, there being a considerable variability among species. The number of parabronchi in both lungs of a Chicken (*Gallus gallus*) is about 300 to 500.[14] The length of the parabronchi within the lungs of a given animal appears to be roughly equal.

From the parabronchial lumen radiates a network of very fine (some μm in diameter) tubular air capillaries, interposed into the system of blood capillaries. Air capillaries, blood capillaries, and their walls, forming the blood/gas membranes, make up most of the peri-parabronchial tissue, which may be viewed as a gas exchange mantle around the parabronchial tubes. The thickness of this mantle is of the same order of magnitude as the radius of the parabronchial lumen, displaying considerable variability among species. In some orders of birds, the air capillaries are functionally blind-ending tubes, and adjacent parabronchi are thus well delimited; whereas in others, the air capillaries of neighboring parabronchi interconnect. Significant convective gas movement, however, through these communicating air capillaries is not expected, since there probably is little pressure difference between adjoining parabronchi.

The avian lungs are compact, small structures which cannot be subdivided macroscopically into subunits such as lobes. They occupy the dorsal portion of the thoracic cavity, and are limited ventrally by a membrane composed mainly of connective tissue, the horizontal septum. The horizontal septum contains some muscle fibers originating from the ribs (Mm. costopulmonales; see below). However, the horizontal septum is neither homologous nor functionally equivalent to the mammalian diaphragm.

3. The Air Sacs

In most birds there exist nine air sacs, four paired and one unpaired (Figure 1). Two pairs, the cranial and caudal thoracic air sacs, have well-defined and smooth walls. The unpaired clavicular air sac has a very complex configuration with many diverticula and extensions even into the surrounding bones. The trachea, main bronchi, esophagus, nerves, and muscles traverse this sac. The cervical sacs are small and diverticulated. Care must be taken not to rupture their walls in the course of tracheotomy. The abdominal air sacs occupy the space between the intestinal loops, and their maximum capacity exceeds by far their actual volume under normal conditions.

The air sacs are usually divided into two groups according to their bronchial connections. The cranial group (cervical, clavicular, and cranial thoracic air sacs) connects to the ventrobronchi, while the sacs of the caudal group (caudal thoracic and abdominal air sacs) have direct communication with the main bronchus. The laterobronchus to the caudal thoracic air sac departs from the main bronchus opposite to the origins of the large, cranial dorsobronchi, while the main bronchus itself opens caudal to the lung into the abdominal sac.

4. Neopulmo vs. Paleopulmo

The features of the respiratory system so far described, and schematically represented in Figure 1, have been found to be present in all birds investigated.[7] Duncker[7] has proposed the term ''paleopulmo'' for this basic arrangement of the lung with parabronchi extending exclusively between ventrobronchi and dorsobronchi. It is the only arrangement occurring in penguins and emus.

In all other birds (which have been studied) an additional network of parabronchi, the neopulmo, is developed, to varied degrees, which extends from the main bronchus and dorsobronchi to the caudal air sacs, entering particularly into their bronchial connections. The neopulmonic parabronchi are laterally apposed to the main bronchus and dorsobronchi. In song birds and fowl-like birds, the neopulmo is particularly well developed. In ducks, the modest development of the neopulmo allows direct access to the dorsobronchi from the lateral body wall. Unlike the situation in the paleopulmo, the parabronchi in the neopulmo form a meshwork. Aside from that, the histologic structure of both types of parabronchi appears to be identical.

In the schema presented above, neopulmonic parabronchi would originate only from dorsobronchi and from the main bronchus. However, with highly developed neopulmo (e.g., in fowl-like and song birds) there exist also some parabronchial connections with ventrobronchi.

B. Ventilation of the Respiratory System
1. Ventilatory Changes in Airway Volume

Inspired air moves into the respiratory system as a result of the expansion of the thoracoabdominal cavity, which is executed by the inspiratory muscles; and during expiration, air is expelled by the action of expiratory muscles. To this extent, the situation is not basically different from that in mammals. But the parabronchial lung appears to undergo only small volume changes in the respiratory cycle. Recent measurements suggest that the parabronchial tissue is distensible so that changes in parabronchial volume might be expected with changing volume of the thoracoabdominal cavity in the course of the respiratory cycle.[15] However, such changes appear to be counteropposed by the phasic activity of the costopulmonary muscles which connect the ribs with the horizontal septum.[16] It appears thus as a justified approximation to view the air sacs as bellows which provide the tidal air flow, part of which is directed through the essentially rigid parabronchial lung.

Earlier authors contended that only the caudal air sacs were ventilated to a significant degree.[17,18] More recent investigations agree, however, that all air sacs are effectively ventilated, the ratio of ventilation to volume being similar in all air sacs.[19-23] Scheid et al.[23] have, moreover, estimated functional volumes and ventilation of the various air sacs in the Duck, using inert gases of low solubility. Further studies have revealed incomplete mixing of inspired gas with residual gas in the air sacs.[24] This finding is of importance in the analysis of the overall gas exchange in birds.

2. Airflow Pathways in the Respiratory Tract: Indirect Evidence

Air reaches the alveoli of mammalian lungs after passing through a number of branching bronchiolar tubes, the airways thus forming a dead-end, to-and-fro system for air flow. The flow of air in the avian lung, on the other hand, cannot easily be predicted from structural considerations. Since the parabronchial lung is open at both ends, air can flow through it in either direction, and the path taken by the air between trachea and the air sac is likewise unpredictable. In fact, this problem has long been a matter of controversy and imaginative speculation (reviewed by Brackenbury in Chapter 2, Biggs and King,[25] King and Farner,[26] King,[10] Bretz and Schmidt-Nielsen,[22] and Scheid[27]).

The theory of Zeuthen[18] appears at first sight to be the most plausible. He regarded the assemblage of the parabronchial tubes (of the paleopulmo) to be in parallel to the main bronchus and thus postulated alternating flow direction through the lung, from ventrobronchi to dorsobronchi during inspiration, and in the opposite direction during expiration. The lung and the main bronchus were assumed to share ventilation in accordance with their relative flow resistance. This theory has received little attention. In fact, authors before and after Zeuthen assumed that air passed through the lung in only one direction, from dorsobronchi to ventrobronchi, either in inspiration or in expiration or in both.

All hypotheses were based on indirect experiments and observations. Distribution of inhaled particles were observed;[17,28-32] gas partial pressures in the air sacs were compared with those in arterial blood;[17-20,31,33-36] normal breathing was compared with breathing through a transected humerus;[25] or the flow pattern was observed in structural models of the respiratory tract.[32,37] More recently, James et al.[38] and Burns et al.[39] employed various radiographic and X-ray techniques to study air movements in the respiratory tract. Controversial results were obtained, and even with agreement in results, conclusions would often differ according to the conceptual models utilized.

Inspiration

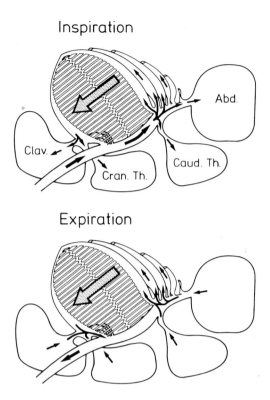

Expiration

FIGURE 2.   Representation of air flow in the respiratory
tract of birds during both phases of ventilation. (Modified
from Scheid.[27])

3. Airflow Pathway: Direct Measurements

More recently, several investigators attempted to measure airflow in the avian respiratory
tract by direct techniques. Bretz and Schmidt-Nielsen[22,40] devised a flow-sensitive catheter
probe of two configurations, incorporating two thermistors as sensing elements. A straight
probe could be inserted directly into the main bronchus, and a curved probe could be advanced
through the main bronchus into a ventrobronchus or dorsobronchus. They observed flow in
awake Ducks during rest and thermal panting as well as in anesthetized birds. Scheid and
Piiper[41,42] devised a flowmeter tube, containing a heat source and a thermocouple element
to be implanted through the lateral body wall into the larger dorsobronchi of the Duck.
Recordings were made in awake animals at rest and during heat-induced panting and also
in pump-ventilated birds after pharmacological muscle relaxation. Brackenbury[43] implanted
small tubes in which flow could be measured manometrically through the lateral body wall
into the major dorsobronchi in Geese and observed airflow in anesthetized, spontaneously
breathing animals.

All these authors observed air to flow in the dorsobronchi during both inspiration and
expiration, flow direction being the same in these bronchi in both respiratory phases, viz.,
from the main bronchus into the dorsobronchi. The anatomy of the bronchial connections
implies that airflow through the parabronchi of the paleopulmo is also in the same direction
during inspiration and expiration, from dorsobronchi towards ventrobronchi (Figure 2). This
pattern is usually referred to as unidirectional airflow. These authors have thus, in respect
of parabronchial flow direction, confirmed the hypothesis first propounded by Bethe.[44]

Support for the unidirectional flow thesis was also obtained by observation of test gases
at various sites in the respiratory system after bolus injections of the gases at key sites.[20,21,45]

Although the unidirectional flow through the parabronchi was thus demonstrated beyond reasonable doubt, there remained controversies about the pattern of flow in other parts of the respiratory system. In particular, direction of inspiratory flow across the ventrobronchial orifices into the main bronchus was much debated, ranging from flow into ventrobronchi,[17,18,37,46,47] flow into the main bronchus,[32] to no flow at all.[20,29,33,36,44] Of particular interest was the "inspired loop hypothesis" of Hazelhoff[32] by which parabronchial gas was supposed to flow more than once over the parabronchi during inspiration. Recent mass spectrometric measurements of the partial pressure profiles for CO_2 and O_2 in the main bronchus and the ventrobronchi of the spontaneously breathing Duck, led to the conclusion that there was no flow across the ventrobronchial orifices during inspiration.[48]

Debate has also been about whether on expiration all flow from caudal air sacs is directed into the (paleopulmonic) lung or whether some gas passes the direct way out through the main bronchus. The best evidence to date suggests that this flow bypassing the lungs is small if not negligible.[22,48]

Airflow through the (paleopulmonic) airways of the resting bird, according to the results outlined above, is schematically represented in Figure 2.

4. Mechanisms Involved in Rectifying Lung Airflow

The simplest explanation for the unidirectional airflow would be the existence of anatomic valves, opened and closed in phase with breathing. Although claimed by a number of authors in the past,[17,28,33,44,46,49] the existence of valves or similar anatomical elements that would cause unidirectional airflow could not be demonstrated by anatomical techniques.[50]

Sequential filling and emptying of the air sacs would be another potential mechanism. In contrast to earlier observations (reviewed by Bretz and Schmidt-Nielsen[22]), small pressure differences appear to exist between the cranial and caudal air sacs, as a result of differences in the time constants for emptying and filling of the sacs, and they play a role in the rectification of flow.[51] According to Brackenbury[52] the cranial air sacs are responsible for driving air flow in the caudocranial direction through the lung during inspiration, while the caudal air sacs determine the flow direction during expiration.

Scheid et al.[47] have shown that the unidirectional dorsobronchial flow persists in the paralyzed, pump-ventilated, and even in the dead animal. Even isolated parts of the bronchial system, excised from an animal that was fixed by glutaraldehyde, showed partial flow rectification or direction-dependent airflow resistance. They concluded that some structure-specific aerodynamic mechanisms were involved. In particular, the Bernoulli effect, boundary layer detachment, and local jet formation were supposed to play a role. Similarly, Brackenbury[53] concluded from his experiments that aerodynamic mechanisms were involved in the rectification of respiratory flow.

Molony et al.[54] found airflow resistance across the ventrobronchial orifices into the main bronchus to be dependent on P_{CO_2} in air, being high at low P_{CO_2}, and vice versa. The anatomic correlate of such a P_{CO_2}-dependent flow resistance was not identified. The authors suggested that this dependence could contribute to functional rectification of flow.

5. Significance of Unidirectional Flow

It is tempting to assume that the unidirectional flow in the parabronchi is of benefit for gas exchange with blood. This would in fact be the case if the parabronchial lung operated as a counter-current system as was proposed earlier.[55] The actual arrangement, however, of blood and gas flow in the parabronchi suggests a different model for gas exchange, the cross-current, the efficiency of which does not depend on the direction of flow (see below). Thus rectification of parabronchial gas flow is not required for the functioning of the gas exchange system.

Piiper and Scheid[56] have suggested that flow reversal would create a functional breath-holding situation during the time required for flow reversal. They have indicated that the rates of drop in P_{O_2} and rise in P_{CO_2} could be intolerably high due to the small parabronchial gas volume. However, direct evidence shows that gas exchange with intermittent ventilatory flow is only slightly impaired compared with gas exchange during continuous ventilatory flow, probably because parabronchial gas is mixed during breath-holding with that in the adjoining airways by way of convection and diffusion. Hence, the functional residual volume in the gas exchange region appears to be larger than the parabronchial volume.[57,58]

During panting, airflow in the dorsobronchi, and thus in the lung, is still unidirectional.[22,42] In fact, the oscillations in flow rate within a respiratory cycle appear to be greatly attenuated at high breathing rates. Reversal of flow at the extremely high respiratory rates during panting could indeed be detrimental, as suggested by Piiper and Scheid.[56]

It is interesting to note that intrapulmonary CO_2 receptors seem to be located at the caudal (inflow) end of the parabronchus;[59] (see References 60 and 61). At this location, the receptors are exposed to a rather low P_{CO_2} where their sensitivity curve is steep. Reversal of flow, on the other hand, would raise the P_{CO_2} in their microenvironment and would possibly shift the receptors into an unfavorable sensitivity range.

It is important to consider that all the above hypotheses and experimental evidence concerned the major, paleopulmonic, compartment of the avian lungs. In the neopulmonic parabronchi (see above) the airflow has to reverse direction from inspiration to expiration from anatomical constraints. In the Duck, in which the neopulmo is moderately developed, the neopulmonic gas exchange has been estimated at about 15% of the total pulmonary gas exchange.[62] The increased development of the neopulmo in the progressive songbirds seems to indicate that the unidirectionality of airflow in the parabronchi is not essential for achieving efficient gas exchange.

III. TRANSPORT OF GASES BY BLOOD

Quantifying gas exchange and its limitations requires accurate data on the transport properties of gases in blood. For the respiratory gases O_2 and CO_2, these are mainly determined by the chemical properties of hemoglobin (Hb), its reversible O_2-binding and buffer properties, and can be described by the blood dissociation curves, i.e., the plots of content vs. partial pressure for O_2 or CO_2. Since the physicochemical properties of vertebrate hemoglobins are similar, differences in the O_2 and CO_2 transport characteristics between birds and mammals are more quantitative than qualitative.

The physiology of gas transport by blood will only be briefly reviewed here; for more detailed discussion and more complete literature, the reader may consult recent reviews.[27,63]

A. Oxygen

Figure 3 shows O_2 dissociation curves for Duck blood at three different levels of pH. The S-shape is typical for O_2 binding to avian as to mammalian Hb. The half-saturation pressure in bird blood, P_{50}, is higher in many birds than in man, but part of the difference results from a negative correlation of P_{50} with body mass.[64] The low affinity of avian blood requires comparatively high P_{O_2} values for full saturation of Hb in avian blood.[65]

The cooperativity between the functional Hb subunits for O_2 binding, which is quantitated by Hill's coefficient, n, has been measured in several species[65] (cf. Reference 27). Of particular interest are the high values of n, exceeding the conventionally accepted theoretical limit of 4, which have been observed in the Chicken[65] and in the Duck,[66] particularly in the high range of O_2 saturation (S_{O_2}).

A number of factors affect O_2 affinity in avian Hb, including H^+ concentration, temperature, and some organic phosphate compounds. The organic phosphate, myoinositol 1,3,4,5,6-pentaphosphate, IPP,[67,68] is the most important agent to decrease O_2 affinity in avian blood.

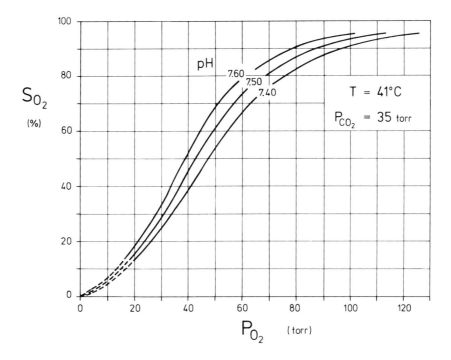

FIGURE 3.   Oxygen dissociation curve of Duck blood at three different pH values. Constructed from data of Scheipers et al.[73] and Meyer et al.[71] (From Scheid, P., *Rev. Physiol. Biochem. Pharmacol.*, 86, 137, 1979. With permission.)

In fact, chicken hemoglobin stripped of IPP shows a P_{50} of less than 3 torr, compared with more than 40 torr in whole blood.[69] The organic phosphate, 2,3-diphosphoglycerate (2,3-DPG), which is the major phosphate of mammalian red cells, does not occur in significant quantities in blood of adult birds. The IPP concentration seems to be constant under most physiologic conditions,[70] and the effect IPP exerts on affinity appears to be saturated at normal IPP levels.

The Bohr effect, i.e., the reduction of O_2 affinity with decreased pH, occurs in avian as it does in mammalian blood.[27] In whole blood, CO_2 does not appear to affect the O_2 affinity other than by way of changing H^+ concentration.[65,71] Because the combination of O_2 with Hb is an exothermic reaction, increased temperature diminishes O_2 affinity. This may be quantified by the temperature coefficient, $\Delta\log(P_{50})/\Delta T$.

B. Carbon Dioxide

The CO_2 equilibrium is represented by the CO_2 dissociation curve (Figure 4), the shape of which appears to be qualitatively similar to that of mammals.[72] Most of the CO_2 content in whole blood is bicarbonate, HCO_3^-. Variation of HCO_3^- with P_{CO_2} is made possible by the presence of buffering substances, mainly the Hb molecule. The contribution of carbamino CO_2 to the CO_2 dissociation curve is not known. The buffer value is similar to that of mammalian blood with similar hemoglobin concentration.[72,73]

Interaction between O_2 and H^+ in binding to Hb constitutes the main reason for the right-shift of the CO_2 dissociation curve with increased O_2 saturation. This Haldane effect is of similar magnitude in avian to that in mammalian blood.

C. Effective Dissociation Curves

The dissociation curves of Figures 3 and 4 represent standard curves in that they pertain to constant P_{CO_2} and pH (Figure 3) or constant O_2 saturation (Figure 4). In vivo, these

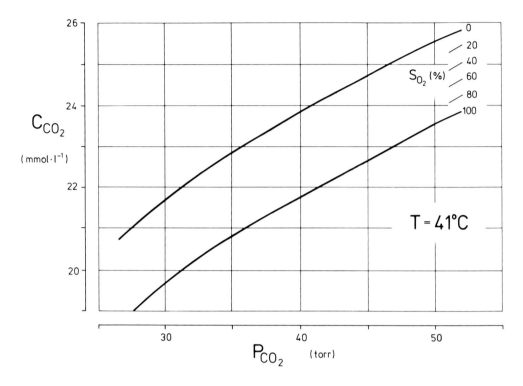

FIGURE 4. Carbon dioxide dissociation curve of Duck blood. After Scheipers et al.[73] (From Scheid, P., *Rev. Physiol. Biochem. Pharmacol.*, 86, 137, 1979. With permission.)

parameters vary as blood circulates through the tissue or lung capillaries. Due to the interaction among CO_2, H^+, and O_2 in Hb binding, expressed by the Bohr and Haldane effects, the variations of O_2 and CO_2 contents in blood in vivo are represented by effective dissociation curves. Scheipers et al.[73] have constructed effective O_2 and CO_2 dissociation curves using arterial blood gas values of resting Chickens and Ducks.[74] These curves are steeper than the standard curves, which is advantageous for gas exchange both in tissues and in the lung.

IV. GAS EXCHANGE IN LUNGS: CROSS-CURRENT MODEL

A. Cross-Current vs. Counter-Current Model

The presence of higher Po_2 in arterial blood as compared to exhaled water is a common observation in fish, where together with anatomical evidence, it forms the basis for the counter-current system as the model adequate for gas exchange in the secondary lamellae (respiratory surface) of fish gills (cf. Reference 75). In this system, blood and water flow in opposite direction in the region where gas exchange takes place. Gas transfer results in a continuous decline of Po_2 in water and a corresponding increase in blood, during the passage through the contact region. In general, this results in an overlap of water and blood Po_2 (and Pco_2) ranges, and at optimum conditions this overlap may be complete: arterial equal to inspired partial pressure, $Pa = PI$, and venous equal to expired partial pressure, $Pv = PE$. With all other pertinent variables identical, the counter-current system obviously provides a higher gas exchange efficiency than the alveolar-type system in that, as a result of the overlap, Po_2 and Pco_2 in arterial blood can come closer to the values in inspired medium.

The structural arrangement of airflow and blood flow in the avian parabronchus is more complex than in fish gills, and it is not easy to derive support for the appropriate type of

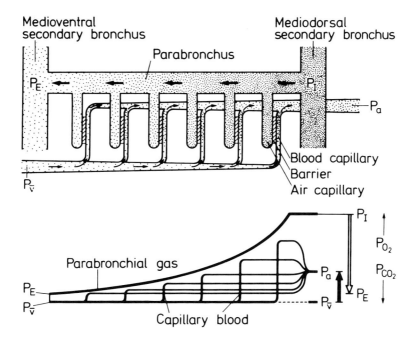

FIGURE 5. Cross-current model for avian parabronchial gas exchange. Above, schema of parabronchus with radially departing air capillaries, and with blood capillaries running from the periphery towards the lumen of the parabronchus and contacting air capillaries of only a small fraction of the parabonchial length. Below, partial pressure profile in the gas phase, from initial-parabronchial (P_I) to end-parabronchial values (P_E); and in blood of the capillaries, arterial blood (P_a) deriving as a mixture from all capillaries. Arrows to the right show the overlap in gas (open arrow) and blood (closed arrow) partial pressures.

gas exchange system from anatomical evidence alone. However, the hypothesis of counter-current flow arrangement may experimentally be tested by measurement of gas exchange upon experimental reversal of parabronchial airflow, and this has in fact been performed.[47]

These authors have cannulated the trachea and both caudal thoracic air sacs in anesthetized Ducks and have passed a continuous flow of air through the parabronchial lung, either in the direction from ventrobronchi towards dorsobronchi, or in the opposite direction. Partial pressures for O_2 and CO_2 were measured in gas entering and leaving the parabronchial lung as well as in arterial and (mixed) venous blood. The striking result was that these partial pressures remained virtually unaffected by reversal of airflow, a result unexpected if the counter-current model was operative. Moreover, overlap between partial pressures in gas and blood was observed, particularly for CO_2, during both flow directions. These results are not compatible with the counter-current model for avian parabronchial gas exchange.

Based on the microscopic anatomy of the periparabronchial tissue (cf. References 7 to 9) Scheid and Piiper[3] have proposed an alternative model, the serial-multicapillary or cross-current system, which had already been considered by Zeuthen.[18] Whereas the counter-current system would require capillaries which run along the parabronchial axis for a significant fraction of its length, capillaries appear to follow a radial direction, originating from arterioles in the periphery of the periparabronchial tissue mantle to be collected by venules close to the parabronchial lumen. On their paths the blood capillaries intertwine with a meshwork of air capillaries, and this is the site for gas exchange. Each capillary thus obtains gas exchange contact with air capillaries of only a small fraction of the total parabronchial length.

A schema of this arrangement is shown in Figure 5. When air traverses the parabronchial

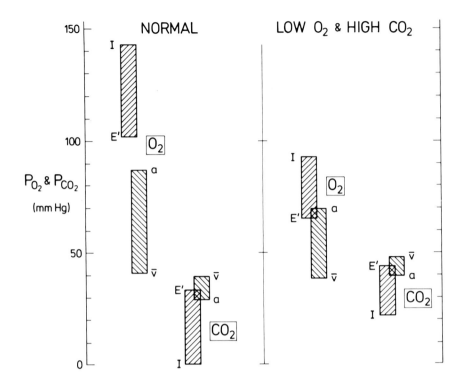

FIGURE 6. Gas-blood CO_2 and O_2 equilibration experimentally observed in the Domestic Fowl. I, E', a, and $\bar{v}$ refer to inspired, end-expired, arterial, and mixed venous P_{CO_2} and P_{O_2} values. The mean differences between $P_{E'}$ and P_a are indicated, their values being negative for gas/blood "overlap". (Data from Piiper, Drees, and Scheid[2] and Scheid and Piiper.[3])

tube, it is continually depleted of O_2 and enriched in CO_2 as it contacts the blood capillaries in serial order. The blood in the blood capillaries, in turn, will be arterialized to varying degrees, depending on their location along the parabronchial tube; the arterialization will be best at the gas inflow end of the parabronchus, and worst at its outflow end. Systemic arterial blood thus constitutes a mixture of blood from all capillaries, and it is easy to conceive that an overlap in gas and blood partial pressures can occur, whereby, e.g., the P_{O_2} in this arterial blood exceeds the P_{O_2} in end-parabronchial gas. Hence, the cross-current model can, like the counter-current system, explain the experimentally observed fact of the gas/blood overlap (Figure 6).

The cross-current system is flow direction-independent. Suppose that airflow is reversed in the system of Figure 5. As a result, the capillary that had been at the inflow end before would now be at the outflow end. This reversal of sequence of capillaries would affect the degree of arterialization of blood in individual capillaries. For the (mixed-) arterial blood, however, no change would occur.

B. Diffusion Limitation in Parabronchial Gas Exchange

In gas exchange organs, two media, viz., air or water and blood, are brought in close contact for transfer of gases. The flow rates determine the transport of respired gases into the region of gas transfer; there is, however, a final path which these gases must traverse without the aid of convective flow. In the avian parabronchial lung, the O_2 molecule has to diffuse from the parabronchial lumen, where it is delivered by the convective flow of parabronchial ventilation, along the gas phase of the air capillary and also across the gas/blood separating tissue membrane (cf. Figure 5).

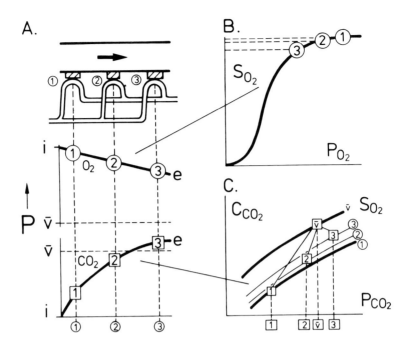

FIGURE 7. Schema to illustrate the peculiar action of the Haldane effect in the parabronchus. In A, the parabronchial gas exchange unit of Figure 5 is represented by three sites, ①, ②, ③, and the values of P_{O_2} and P_{CO_2} at these sites are shown on the corresponding gas P_{O_2} and P_{CO_2} profiles. B represents an O_2 dissociation curve where O_2 saturation, S_{O_2}, in blood (see Figure 3) at the three sites can be read from corresponding P_{O_2} values. (Equality of gas and end-capillary blood partial pressures is assumed at each site.) C represents the CO_2 dissociation curves for different S_{O_2} values (see Figure 4). CO_2 content, C_{CO_2}, is obtained from the P_{CO_2} values at each site and the corresponding S_{O_2} values. It is evident that P_{CO_2} at site ③ exceeds mixed venous P_{CO_2}, although C_{CO_2} in mixed venous blood is higher than in blood at site ③. As a result, P_{CO_2} in end-parabronchial gas (Pe_{CO_2}, site ③) may exceed mixed venous P_{CO_2}, $P\bar{v}_{CO_2}$. (From Scheid, P., *Rev. Physiol. Biochem. Pharmacol.*, 86, 137, 1979. With permission.)

Although the (average) path in the air capillary (a few hundred μm) is much larger than that through the tissue membrane (a fraction of a μm), the diffusion resistance along the air capillaries is probably considerably smaller than that through the membrane. This is due to the fact that the diffusivity in air is some 100,000 times larger than that in water (or tissue).[76] As a result, diffusion in the air capillaries of the parabronchus does not, under normal conditions, impose a serious resistance on overall gas exchange[77] (cf. Reference 27).

C. Haldane Effect and the Particular Enhancement of CO_2 Transfer

In alveolar lungs, the interaction among H^+ and O_2 in binding to Hb, expressed by the Bohr-Haldane effect of blood, results in an increased gas exchange efficiency. This may be quantified by an increase in the slopes of the effective binding curves for O_2 and CO_2, resulting in an increased value for perfusive conductance, G_{perf} (see Section V). This effect operates in the avian as it does in the mammalian lung. However, the Haldane effect may exert a further particular enhancement of CO_2 exchange in the parabronchial lung due to its peculiar structural arrangement.

Figure 7 serves to illustrate the underlying mechanisms. The gas exchange rate of each parabronchial segment depends on the component conductances (see Section V). While the ventilatory conductance G_{vent}, is the same for O_2 and CO_2, G_{perf} and the diffusive conductance, G_{diff}, for CO_2 exceed the respective values for O_2, since CO_2 solubility in tissue is larger, and the dissociation curve is steeper for CO_2 compared with O_2. Thus, in the initial segments CO_2 release will exceed O_2 uptake, while the opposite is true for segments at the outflow end. This is reflected in a steeper gas partial pressure gradient along the parabronchus for CO_2 than for O_2 (Figure 7A). Thus, P_{O_2} in end-capillary blood (which is close to the P_{O_2} in the gas phase of the contacted segment) stays relatively high throughout the parabronchus resulting, by virtue of the flat O_2 dissociation curve at high P_{O_2}, in relatively high O_2 saturation in end-capillary blood throughout (Figure 7B). Figure 7C shows the CO_2 dissociation curves corresponding to O_2 saturation, S_{O_2}, in mixed-venous blood ($\bar{v}$) and in end-capillary blood of the three compartments of Figure 7A. It is evident that end-capillary P_{CO_2} exceeds mixed-venous P_{CO_2}. By virtue of the Haldane effect, CO_2 may thus be released ($C\bar{v}_{CO_2}$ exceeding end-capillary C_{CO_2} at site ③) against an apparent P_{CO_2} gradient (end-capillary P_{CO_2} at site ③ exceeding $P\bar{v}_{CO_2}$).

In the limiting case, when there is no CO_2 release at the end of the parabronchus while O_2 uptake continues, the blood of the last capillary will be oxygenated with no CO_2 release. Hence, P_{CO_2} in blood leaving this capillary will approach oxygenated mixed-venous P_{CO_2} ($P\bar{v}_{CO_2}$) which may be substantially above true mixed-venous P_{CO_2}.[76] The result is that end-parabronchial P_{CO_2}, Pe_{CO_2}, may not only exceed arterial P_{CO_2}, Pa_{CO_2}, as expected from the cross-current arrangement, but also $P\bar{v}_{CO_2}$, as a result of the Haldane effect in concert with this arrangement. Thus, this mechanism constitutes a peculiar enhancement of CO_2 release in the cross-current system.

Zeuthen[18] qualitatively proposed the same mechanism to explain the fact that P_{CO_2} values in expired gas could exceed those in mixed-venous blood. Davies and Dutton[79] and Meyer et al.[78] have recently observed PE'_{CO_2} to exceed $P\bar{v}_{CO_2}$ in the chicken. Meyer et al.[78] have proposed the above mechanisms and have criticized the conclusions of Davies and Dutton,[79] who had invoked the Wien effect as an explanation[1] (cf. Reference 3).

V. QUANTITATIVE ANALYSIS OF GAS EXCHANGE

A. Basic Parameters

The following variables are required for a quantitative description of gas exchange in the avian lung (typical units in brackets). The terminology, the system of units, and the dimensions used are in accordance with Piiper et al.[80] Figure 8 serves to illustrate schematically the meaning of the symbols used:

1. *Transfer rate*, $\dot{M}$, of O_2 and CO_2, i.e., the amounts of these gases exchanged per unit time between the gas phase and the blood (mmol $\cdot$ min^{-1}).

2. *Partial pressure*, P, of O_2 or CO_2 in the gas entering (Pi) and leaving the parabronchus (Pe) and in mixed venous (P$\bar{v}$) and arterial blood (Pa) (torr or kPa).

3. *Capacitance coefficient*, β, defined as the increment in concentration, C, per increment in partial pressure, P, for both the gas and the blood phase [mmol $\cdot \ell^{-1} \cdot$ torr^{-1}]. For gaseous medium and for exclusively physical solution, β is independent of P (constant solubility). In particular, in the gas phase, β_g is identical for all (ideal) gases and is only dependent upon temperature. For 41°C, the body temperature of many experimental birds, $\beta_g = 0.0510$ mmol $\cdot \ell^{-1} \cdot$ torr^{-1}. For physical solution, β equals the solubility coefficient, α. For O_2 and CO_2 in blood, β is dependent on P, and is equal to the slope of the respective dissociation curve.

4. *Flow rate*, $\dot{V}$ and $\dot{Q}$, of parabronchial gas and lung capillary blood [m$\ell \cdot$ min^{-1}]. While $\dot{Q}$ is nearly identical with cardiac output, the parabronchial ventilation is in general smaller than the total ventilation $\dot{V}E$, due to presence of dead space.

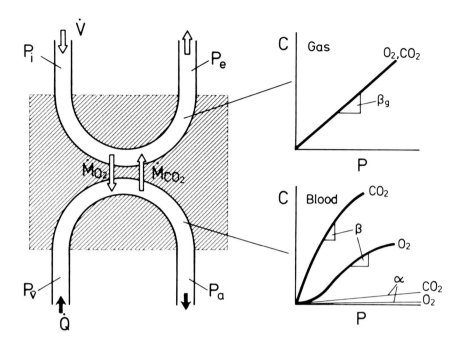

FIGURE 8.   Representation of a gas exchange system to define the important parameters. To the right, plot of concentration, C, against partial pressure, P, in the gas phase (upper) or blood (lower). Slope of these curves represents the solubility coefficient, β. In gas phase $\beta = \beta_g$ is identical for all (ideal) gases. For physical solubility in blood, $\beta = \alpha$, i.e., identical with physical solubility coefficient. See text for details. (From Scheid, P., *Rev. Physiol. Biochem. Pharmacol.*, 86, 137, 1979. With permission.)

5. *Conductance*, G [mmol · min^{-1} · torr^{-1}]. Defined as transfer rate, $\dot{M}$, per driving partial pressure difference, ΔP:

$$G = \dot{M}/\Delta P \tag{1}$$

The mass balance requires for the gas side

$$\dot{M} = \dot{V} \cdot \beta_g \cdot (Pi - Pe) \tag{2}$$

and for blood,

$$\dot{M} = \dot{Q} \cdot \beta_b \cdot (Pa - P\bar{v}) \tag{3}$$

The ventilation and perfusion conductances, G_{vent} and G_{perf}, are easily obtained from Equations 1, 2, and 3:

$$G_{vent} = \dot{V} \cdot \beta_g \tag{4}$$

$$G_{perf} = \dot{Q} \cdot \beta_b \tag{5}$$

For diffusive transport across the blood/gas separating membrane, the diffusive conductance, G_{diff}, may be obtained from Fick's law of diffusion:

$$G_{diff} = K \cdot A/l \qquad (6)$$

where A and l are area and thickness of the membrane, and where Krogh's diffusion constant, K, is dependent on the diffusing gas species, the material of the membrane, and the temperature. G_{diff} is often referred to as the diffusing capacity, D.

For diffusive transport in the gas phase of the air capillaries, Equation 6 applies as well, A and l in this case being (combined) cross-sectional area and length of the air capillary, and $K = d \cdot \beta_g$, where d is the diffusion coefficient of the gas under study in the air capillary gas.

The relationship between the partial pressures in parabronchial gas, Pi and Pe, and in blood, Pa and Pv̄, is determined by the type of the gas exchange system, in our case the cross-current system, and the conductance values, G_{vent}, G_{perf}, and G_{diff}.

Of particular interest is the blood-gas overlap of Po_2 and Pco_2 (see Section IV.A), (Pe − Pa)/(Pi − Pv̄). According to Scheid and Piiper[3] and Piiper and Scheid,[4] the following relationship is valid for the cross-current system.

$$\frac{Pe - Pa}{Pi - P\bar{v}} = 1 - \left(1 + \frac{G_{vent}}{G_{perf}}\right)\left[1 - \exp\left\{-\frac{G_{perf}}{G_{vent}}\left(1 - \exp\left(-\frac{G_{diff}}{G_{perf}}\right)\right)\right\}\right] \qquad (7)$$

The most extensive overlap, i.e., negative values for (Pe − Pa)/(Pi − Pv̄), is attained at high values of G_{diff} and when the G_{vent}/G_{perf} ratio is in the range of 0.1 to 1.0.[4]

The above analysis leading to Equation 7 is valid only for the ideal cross-current system, as it is bound to a number of assumptions, of which the following are the more important.

1. Radial diffusivity, within the parabronchial lumen, and diffusivity along the air capillaries, is infinite. Thus, the air capillaries offer no diffusive resistance to gas transfer.
2. Transport of gases along the parabronchial axis occurs exclusively by convection, diffusivity in this direction being neglected.
3. The system is in steady state, meaning constancy in time of all parameters. In particular, both flow rates, V̇ and Q̇, are assumed to be constant in time, as are the partial pressures Pi and Pv̄.
4. β is constant, independent of P (linear blood dissociation curves).
5. The parabronchial lung is perfectly homogeneous. It may thus be represented by one single parabronchus, which receives all blood and gas flows and is equipped with the total diffusing capacity.

These assumptions will be critically reviewed in the following section, and it will be examined to what extent the ideal cross-current model is applicable to real avian lungs.

B. Limitation of Model Analysis: the Real Parabronchial Lung
1. Axial Diffusion
Crank and Gallagher[81] showed that the partial pressure profiles along the parabronchial axis would be affected by finite axial diffusion, but the effect on gas exchange was insignificant except at unphysiologically low parabronchial flow rates. Qualitatively, axial diffusion results in mixing of intraparabronchial gas, whereby the parabronchus would functionally approach the alveolar pool model and thus lose the elevated gas exchange efficiency of the cross-current system.

2. Radial Diffusion
On the basis of a simplified model, Zeuthen[18] and Hazelhoff[32] estimated the limitation

offered by air capillaries to O_2 and CO_2 exchange to be negligible under all conditions, including flight. Scheid[77] has criticized their model as not correctly reflecting gas exchange in the subelement comprising the air capillary and the blood capillary in contact with it. He reevaluated the air capillary diffusion limitation, using the model shown in Figure 9. It consists of the blind-ending air capillary in gas exchange contact with a blood capillary. According to anatomical evidence,[9] blood flows from the blind end of the air capillary to its origin from the parabronchial lumen. In this model, gas exchange occurs all along the air capillary and concentration gradients may develop along the air capillary. The partial pressure profiles for O_2 in air capillary gas (referred to as stratification) and in blood capillary blood are schematically shown by dashed lines in the absence of gas phase diffusion limitation, and by continuous lines, with finite diffusivity. The equilibration deficit due to gas phase diffusion limitation is represented by the difference between the end-capillary partial pressures in the absence and presence of gas phase diffusion limitation.

Calculations for this and for other models which account for the anatomical evidence presented[9,82,83] suggest that for most conditions the effect of finite gas phase diffusion is small, particularly for resting conditions,[77] and this has been experimentally confirmed.[84] Only at elevated metabolism may air capillary diffusion resistance become rate limiting. There are substantial uncertainties, however, in these estimates since morphometric data needed in these calculations are incomplete. Crank and Gallagher[81] have performed similar calculations with similar results.

3. Steady-State Conditions

It was assumed in the model of Section V.A that at any given site in the parabronchus all variables that determine gas exchange are constant in time. These "independent" variables include conductances, composition of inspired air, mixed venous blood gases, and metabolic rate. Evidently both $\dot{V}$ and $\dot{Q}$ vary with time in the respiratory and cardiac cycles. Very little is known about pulsatile blood flow in the pulmonary capillary bed, but experimental investigations exist on the implications of nonsteady parabronchial gas flow.

In calculating alveolar gas exchange, the gas flow rate is usually considered to be constant since the large ratio of residual to tidal volume results in an effective buffering of the cyclic gas flow rates, resulting in only minor variations of alveolar gas composition in phase with tidal volume (e.g., Piiper and Scheid[1]). In birds, the situation is different, since the parabronchial gas volume is much smaller on the tidal volume scale[8] whereby significant changes in parabronchial gas composition are expected to occur.[56] Scheid et al.[57] found, however, no significant impairment of O_2 exchange when parabronchial flow was oscillated at rates at or above naturally occurring respiratory rates. The effective parabronchial gas volume estimated on the basis of the experimental data was about twice the anatomic value.[8] Mixing of parabronchial gas with gas in the adjoining larger bronchi may explain part of this apparent discrepancy. Thus, variations in parabronchial gas flow do not appear to seriously limit applicability of the cross-current model.

However, tidal ventilation together with the airflow pattern in the respiratory system are responsible for cyclic variations in the initial-parabronchial partial pressures (Pi) both for O_2 and CO_2. In inspiration, dead space gas enters the parabronchi first, followed by fresh gas; while during expiration, gas entering the parabronchi derives from caudal air sacs.[24] Scheid et al.[85] and Geiser et al.[86] have used a flow-weighted mean value for Pi in their calculations using the cross-current model. Thus, there is a substantial variation in Pi within the respiratory cycle and its implication on parabronchial gas exchange is not precisely known. It is interesting to note that variations of end-parabronchial gas composition within the respiratory cycle appear to be small.[48]

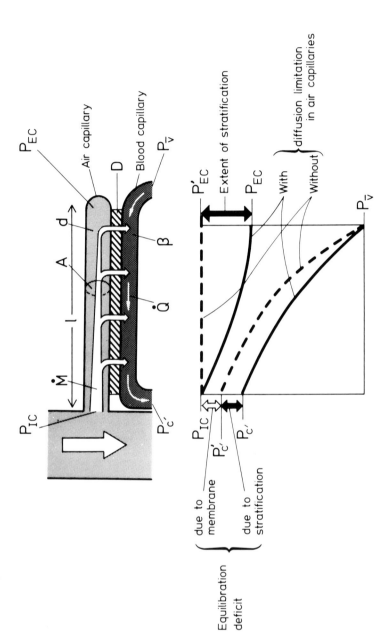

FIGURE 9.   Stratification in avian air capillaries. An air capillary, of length, l, and cross-sectional area, A, is shown to originate radially from the parabronchial lumen. A blood capillary contacts this air capillary in its course from the periphery towards the parabronchial lumen, both capillaries being separated by a tissue membrane of diffusing capacity, DM. Arrow in parabronchial lumen denotes gas flow direction; arrow in air capillary, O_2 transport, $\dot{M}$ (by diffusion); arrows in flow, direction of blood perfusion, $\dot{Q}$; PIC, PEC, partial pressures in gas at the origin and the end of air capillary; Pv̄, Pc′, partial pressures in mixed venous and end-capillary blood. The diagram below shows partial pressure profiles in gas and blood with finite (continuous curves) or negligible (dashed curves) diffusion resistance in the gas phase of the air capillaries (realized, e.g., by infinite diffusivity, d), for which case P′EC denotes partial pressure in the gas at the end of the air capillary, and P′c′, in blood at the end of the blood capillary. Calculations are based on those morphometrical data which are most unfavorable for diffusion. (From Scheid, P., *Rev. Physiol. Biochem. Pharmacol.,* 86, 137, 1979. With permission.)

4. Linear Dissociation Curves

The effective solubility, β_b, was assumed to be constant, independent of partial pressure. This is strictly true for inert gases. For CO_2 and O_2, however, chemical reaction occurs as reflected in nonlinear blood dissociation curves, and β_b does vary with partial pressure (see Figures 3 and 4). In the parabronchial lung, blood partial pressures span a range from $P\bar{v}$ to the end-capillary value of the first blood capillary at the gas inflow end, which is close to Pi. Over this range, β_b must essentially be constant, i.e., straight dissociation curve, for the equations to be applicable.

For O_2 in normoxia, this condition is certainly not met. In hypoxia, however, the dissociation curve is steeper, hence, the range of blood P_{O_2} values more narrow; also, the curve is more straight in this range. Therefore, the assumption of constant β_b for O_2 is better met in hypoxia. Analogous arguments apply for CO_2.

The effects of the curvilinearity of the dissociation curves are different for O_2 and CO_2 (see Reference 27). For O_2, the curvature in the normoxic range results in maintaining a large gas-blood partial pressure difference and, thus, a large pressure head for diffusion across the gas-blood separating tissue membrane. Thus, the curvilinearity enhances the efficiency of pulmonary gas exchange, and this is true for the parabronchial lung as well as for the alveolar lung. For CO_2, the curvature of the dissociation curve is functionally opposed to that of O_2.

In alveolar lungs, the effects of curvilinear dissociation curves may be accounted for by the Bohr integration procedure (e.g., Piiper and Scheid[1]) which, although applicable, is tedious when used for the cross-current model. Alternatively, experimental hypoxia combined with hypercapnia may be used for a quantitative gas exchange analysis.[3,84]

5. Inhomogeneities

Gas exchange in the ideal parabronchus depends on three conductances: G_{vent}, G_{perf}, and G_{diff}. If these parameters are known, the output partial pressures, Pe and Pa, can be determined using Equations 2 to 7 for any set of input partial pressures, Pi and $P\bar{v}$; or, $P\bar{v}$ can be determined for given Pi and $\dot{M}$. In fact, only two ratios of these conductances need to be known, e.g., $X = G_{vent}/G_{perf}$ and $Y = G_{diff}/G_{perf}$ (cf. Reference 4). If these conductance ratios are constant between parabronchi or within each parabronchus, i.e., when G_{vent} and G_{diff} are equally distributed to G_{perf}, the parabronchial lung may be said to be functionally homogeneous. Functional heterogeneity thus implies regional differences in the conductance ratios.

Evidently, regional heterogeneity can exist between parabronchi and may be termed "parallel heterogeneity" (Figure 10B). Here, $\dot{V}$, $\dot{Q}$, and D are different between parabronchi in such a way that either G_{vent}/G_{perf} or G_{diff}/G_{perf} or both differ. But also within the subunit elements of a given parabronchus there may exist heterogeneity, termed "series heterogeneity" (Figure 10B). Since $\dot{V}$ is (nearly) constant along the parabronchus, it is only G_{diff} that can be unevenly alotted to G_{perf} to create the series heterogeneity of G_{diff}/G_{perf}.

The various heterogeneity effects have been investigated in some detail by Powell and Wagner[87,88] and reviewed by Powell and Scheid.[89] The general conclusions are series and parallel heterogenities reduce gas exchange efficiency of a cross-current gas exchange system. The effects are increased with small β_b and high G_{diff}. The reduced gas exchange efficiency can be described as a combined blood shunt (venous admixture) and air shunt (inspired admixture, dead space).

Direct evidence for heterogeneities by measuring $\dot{V}$, $\dot{Q}$, and D separately within or between parabronchi is difficult. Injection of labeled microspheres into the blood stream has been used to determine the blood flow distribution within the lung.[90-93] There appears to be a slight decrease in specific blood flow along the parabronchus from the mediodorsal (inspiratory) to the medioventral (expiratory) end, and this does not seem to be due to O_2 depletion

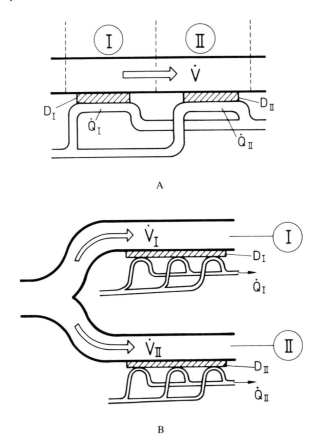

FIGURE 10. Schematic representation of series (A) and parallel in-
homogeneities (B), illustrated on a simplified two-compartment system
(compartments I and II). Further explanation in the text. (From Scheid,
P., *Rev. Physiol. Biochem. Pharmacol.*, 86, 137, 1979. With
permission.)

in parabronchial gas towards the expiratory end.[90] Since no measurements are available on
the distribution of D along the parabronchus, it is not known to what extent this inequality
of $\dot{Q}$ constitutes a series heterogeneity.

To estimate parallel heterogeneity, Burger et al.[84] have used a two-compartment model
like that of Figure 10B in the analysis of O_2 and CO_2 exchange in the Duck. On the assumption
that D for CO_2 is infinite, they estimated the degree of parallel maldistribution from CO_2
exchange and calculated D for O_2 by accounting for this heterogeneity.

Use of inert gases bears particular advantages in the analysis of gas exchange, mainly
due to two factors. First, inert gases are not chemically bound in blood, and hence, β_b is
constant and equal to physical solubility, α, whereby problems due to nonlinear dissociation
curves do not exist. Second, inert gases are not expected to be diffusion limited because
their $D/(\dot{Q}\beta_b)$ ratio is much larger than that for O_2 or CO_2, for which β_b is enlarged by
chemical binding (cf. Reference 1). Hence, inert gas transfer is affected only by parallel
G_{vent}/G_{perf} inequalities.

Burger et al.[84] have used the high-solubility gas diethyl ether to estimate ventilation of
unperfused parabronchi, but a more rigorous analysis has recently been performed by Powell
and Wagner.[87] These authors have used the multiple inert gas elimination method that was

developed by Wagner, West, and their colleagues for the alveolar lung (cf. Reference 94). In this technique, transfer of a number of inert gases of widely differing solubility is measured and used to determine the unknown ventilation and perfusion in a great number (e.g., 50) of parallel lung units (e.g., parabronchi).

In anesthetized, spontaneously breathing or pump-ventilated Geese[88] the distribution of $\dot{V}$ and $\dot{Q}$ to compartments with different $\dot{V}/\dot{Q}$ was estimated. This distribution allowed calculation of arterial and mixed-venous P_{O_2} and P_{CO_2} values for the experimental animal. The agreement between predicted and measured values was fairly good, particularly for CO_2. For O_2, however, Pa was consistently lower than predicted indicating that, aside from parallel heterogeneities, there were other factors depressing the gas exchange efficiency which were not taken into account. The effect may well have been due to diffusion limitation, particularly across the blood/gas separating tissue membrane (where K for O_2 is much less than for CO_2).

6. Gas Exchange in Neopulmo

Presence of neopulmonic parabronchi in addition to the paleopulmonic parabronchi in most birds may be regarded as a special type of heterogeneity. Neopulmonic parabronchi are essentially in series between the trachea and caudal air sacs. Hence, the direction of gas flow in them changes in the respiratory cycle, and they can affect the composition of gas entering paleopulmonic parabronchi during expiration. This could lead to a type of series heterogeneity, but it has not been fully investigated to date. Duncker[8] has suggested that neopulmo, when sufficiently developed, might constitute the predominant or exclusive site for gas exchange at rest, whereas paleopulmonic parabronchi would contribute significantly only during increased O_2 demand, particularly in exercise. Experimental evidence supporting this view has not been found.[90,95] (See Reference 27.)

C. Determination of Diffusing Capacity

For the homogeneous cross-current model in steady state and with constant β_b (linear blood gas dissociation curve) the diffusing capacity D ($= G_{diff}$) is obtained by combining Equations 2 to 5 and 7 (see Reference 27):

$$D = -\frac{\dot{M}}{Pa - P\overline{v}} \cdot \ln\left\{ 1 + \frac{Pa - P\overline{v}}{Pi - Pe} \cdot \ln\left(\frac{Pe - P\overline{v}}{Pi - P\overline{v}}\right)\right\} \qquad (8)$$

It was shown above that D_{O_2} should be measured in hypoxia to reduce effects of lung heterogeneity and of alinear O_2 dissociation curves.

For calculation of D_{O_2} according to Equation 8, O_2 uptake rate, $\dot{M}$, has to be measured together with partial pressures in blood, Pa and $P\overline{v}$, and in parabronchial gas, Pi and Pe. $\dot{M}$ can rather easily be measured, particularly when expired gas is measured. For measurement of Pa, any peripheral artery may be punctured, but for $P\overline{v}$, a blood sample has to be collected from the right ventricle or, preferably, the pulmonary artery. Initial- and end-parabronchial gas are not easily accessible for measurement of Pi and Pe. A valid approximation to Pe may be obtained in cranial air sac gas, since Powell et al.[48] have shown that composition of gas in medioventral secondary bronchi does not fluctuate significantly in the respiratory cycle and is very close to that in the clavicular air sac. Composition of initial-parabronchial gas, collected, e.g., in the dorsobronchi, does, however, exhibit cyclic variations in the breathing cycle.[48] During early inspiration, dead space gas is reinhaled, followed by fresh gas. During expiration, it is caudal air sac gas that determines Pi. The time-averaged Pi value may be close to that of caudal air sac which may thus be used as an approximation in the calculation of D according to Equation 8 (see Reference 86).

Burger et al.[84] have used a special ventilatory technique, unidirectional ventilation, whereby gas is insufflated into the caudal air sacs at a constant rate, made to flow across the parabronchi, and to leave via the trachea. With this technique, initial- and end-parabronchial gas composition is constant in time and can easily be measured. They have determined D_{O_2} in the (anesthetized) Duck to average $0.1 \text{ mmol} \cdot \text{min}^{-1} \cdot \text{torr}^{-1}$. Measured D_{O_2} was smaller when hypoxia was less severe reflecting the larger effects of lung heterogeneity in normoxia compared with hypoxia (cf. assumption of constant β_b). The somewhat smaller values for D_{O_2} in the Chicken[3] and the Duck[86] are most likely due to the fact that experimental conditions in these studies were less appropriate for measurement of D_{O_2}.

Abdalla et al.[96] have recently reported morphometric data obtained from lungs of the Domestic Fowl from which they estimated lung diffusing capacity. Their value was well in the range of the physiologic estimates in the Chicken.[3] Similarly, the morphometric estimate of D_{O_2} in the Mallard, *Anas platyrhynchos*,[97] compared well with the physiologic estimate in the Muscovy Duck, *Cairina moschata*.[84] Similar estimates were obtained in other birds.[98] As Abdalla et al.[96] correctly discuss, comparison of morphometric with physiologic estimates of lung diffusing capacity calls for caution (see Reference 99). This is because the physiologic value depends critically on a number of functional parameters and measurements that are inaccessible to the morphometrist. Among these are the possible functional heterogeneities in respect of ventilation, perfusion, and diffusing capacity; the diffusive properties of the gases in tissues or blood; and possible limitations by chemical reaction in blood. Since some of these parameters are unknown, and their estimates could thus be wrong in either direction, it is not even safe to assume that the morphometric estimate of lung diffusing capacity constitutes an upper limit for its physiological counterpart. Thus, while at given lung ventilation and perfusion the physiologic D_{O_2} is a measure for the lung potential to transfer gases, the morphometric estimate constitutes a parameter to indicate the mean area-to-thickness ratio of the gas exchanging surface.

VI. RESPIRATION AND GAS EXCHANGE UNDER VARIOUS CONDITIONS

A. Rest

In Table 1 we have compiled literature data on respiration and gas exchange in a number of domestic birds at rest. These values were obtained in unrestrained, or lightly restrained, animals in which a fairly complete set of parameters could be measured.

In estimating the extent to which these data represent normal values of unrestrained animals, arterial P_{CO_2} constitutes a sensitive measure, since any change in ventilation, e.g., hyperventilation in excitement or hypoventilation with central depression by anesthesia, will be reflected in changing Pa_{CO_2}. Normal values of Pa_{CO_2} in the freely running Hen and Duck have been measured by Kawashiro and Scheid[74] who used remote-controlled techniques for blood sampling.[100] Their mean values of 33 torr for the Hen and 38 torr for the Muscovy Duck compare favorably with the range of values in Table 1, suggesting that these parameters are indeed close to normal values.

Most of the data in Table 1 show only quantitative differences from reported values for mammals. They could be explained in part by body mass (M_B) differences (cf. References 101 to 103).

B. Elevated Metabolism

For proper appreciation of the capacity and limitations of the gas exchange system, it is best studied under such stress as exercise, environmental hypoxia, or cold. This is particularly true for birds which, on their long-range flight, simultaneously face a number of these stresses, viz., long-lasting exercise at high altitude with potential environmental hypoxia and cold. It has, in fact, been proposed that high metabolic rates and environmental hypoxia

Table 1
GAS EXCHANGE VARIABLES IN AWAKE RESTING BIRDS

	Pigeon[123]	Hen[2]	Pekin Duck[162]	Pekin Duck[163]	Muscovy Duck[163]
M_B (kg)	0.38	1.6	2.37	2.4	2.16
$\dot{M}_{O_2}$ (mmol · min^{-1})	0.35	1.09	1.67	—	—
f_{resp} (min^{-1})	27.3	23	15.6	8.2	10.5
V_T (mℓ)	7.5	33	58.5	98	69
V_E (ℓ · min^{-1})	0.204	0.760	0.910	0.807	0.700
$\dot{Q}$ (ℓ · min^{-1})	0.127	0.430	0.423	0.973	0.844
$P_{E'_{O_2}}$ (torr)	—	101.8	—	100.1	96.6
$P_{a_{O_2}}$ (torr)	95	87	100	93.1	96.1
$P_{\bar{v}_{O_2}}$ (torr)	50	40.8	69.3	63.3	55.9
$P_{E'_{CO_2}}$ (torr)	—	33.0	—	34.2	34.2
$P_{a_{CO_2}}$ (torr)	34	29.2	33.8	36.3	35.9
$P_{\bar{v}_{CO_2}}$ (torr)	—	39.3	—	37.3	42.6

Note: Data collected from birds in body plethysmographs except References 2 and 163 which used endotracheal tubes in lightly restrained upright birds. $\dot{M}_{O_2}$ not given for Reference 161 because mixed-expired gases were not measured. M_B, body mass; $\dot{M}_{O_2}$, O_2 uptake rate; f_{resp}, respiratory frequency; V_T, tidal volume; V_E, total ventilation; $\dot{Q}$, cardiac output, $P_{E'}$, P_a, $P_{\bar{v}}$, partial pressures (for O_2 or CO_2) in end-expired air, arterial, or mixed venous blood.

may have been selective pressures for a very efficient gas exchange system in birds.[104,105] Studies on birds under these naturally occurring conditions are extremely difficult, but certain activities can be simulated in the laboratory (e.g., treadmill running, wind tunnel flight, hypoxia) or studied with the use of radiotelemetry.

1. Flight

Flight constitutes the natural exercise of most birds, but measurements of respiratory parameters are scarce. Oxygen uptake of birds on long flights is about twice the maximal value obtained on mammals of comparable size during shorter periods of exercise.[106,107] Measurements have been made on Hummingbirds (*Colibri coruscans*) hovering in an enclosure[108,109] and, by telemetry, on birds during short flights.[110,111] Telemetry from large birds imprinted to fly for longer times behind a moving experimental platform appears to be a promising technique, but so far only heart rate and respiratory frequency, along with wing beat frequency, have been measured.[112]

Investigations on birds trained to fly in a wind tunnel have been particularly valuable.[113] This technique allows rather sophisticated measurement of respiration and gas exchange since the birds are made to fly at a point that does not move relative to the observer and his instruments. Thus, blood and air have been sampled using indwelling cathethers and a face mask.

Table 2 presents a collection of data obtained in flying birds of widely differing body mass. It is due to the difficulties of these experiments that complete gas exchange data are still missing. However, the published data may be used to calculate parameters that are important for gas exchange. One such variable is the effective ventilation, V_{eff}, calculated as total ventilation minus dead space ventilation. This quantity constitutes a reasonable estimate for parabronchial ventilation, V_P, i.e., for ventilation of the gas exchange region.

According to estimates, values of V_P appear to increase at least as much as, or even more than, $\dot{M}_{O_2}$ during flight (Table 2). This would explain the observed increase in P_{O_2}, and

Table 2
GAS EXCHANGE DURING FLIGHT

	Starling[114]		Pigeon[105]		Black Duck[110]	
	Rest	Flight	Rest	Flight	Rest	Flight
M_B (g)	78		380		1,026	
M_{O_2} (mmol $\cdot$ min^{-1})	0.13	1.21	0.37	3.72	0.84	10.58
f_{resp} (min^{-1})	92	180	26	487	27	158
V_T (mℓ)	0.67	2.80	7.2	6.0	30.2	71.0
V_E ($\ell \cdot$ min^{-1})	0.061	0.504	0.188	2.92	0.79	10.83
V_D (mℓ)	0.22		2.2		6.4	
V_{P^a} ($\ell \cdot$ min^{-1})	0.041	0.46	0.13	1.8	0.62	9.8

[a]   Parabronchial ventilation, estimated as the difference between total ventilation, V_E, and dead space ventilation, assuming dead space volume, V_D, equals tracheal volume.

decrease in P_{CO_2}, in the clavicular air sac gas of the flying Starling (*Sturnus vulgaris*).[114] However, blood gases have not been measured in this experiment, and estimates of their changes with exercise are difficult due to the peculiar nature of parabronchial gas exchange. Butler et al.[115] have measured Pa_{CO_2} increasing with flight in the Pigeon (*Columba livia*); at the same time, a significant drop in arterial pH, probably due to lactic acid formation in the exercising flight muscle, was responsible for a fall in arterial O_2 content, by way of the Bohr effect.

2. Walking and Running

Although bird locomotion is typically associated with flight, several avian families primarily rely on bipedal walking and running. Experimentally, running on a treadmill has become a useful method to study cardio-respiratory adjustments to exercise in birds.[116-120] The demand placed on the respiratory system during running can be as large as during flight.

Unfortunately, the number of variables that can be measured in birds on treadmills is limited and all of the crucial variables have not been measured in any one species. Notable is the lack of simultaneous measurements of expired (or clavicular air sac) and arterial P_{O_2}. The most complete data have been collected in the Domestic Hen and Pekin Duck (Table 3).

The maximum increase in metabolism reported for running birds is 12 times the resting value, obtained in domestic cocks running at 2.5 m $\cdot$ sec^{-1}.[121] This value is similar to those reported during flight (see Section VI.B.1). The relative increases in Table 3 are lower than those of Table 2 because the resting values collected on the treadmill before it is turned on are almost twice the "true" resting values because of anticipation (cf. Reference 120). Also, the maximum O_2 consumption during running is less in the Domestic Hen which is slower than the cock, and in the Duck which is an awkward runner. Kiley et al.[116] did not measure O_2 consumption, but Bech and Nomoto[118] ran Pekin Ducks at the same speed, but without the 3° incline used by Kiley et al.,[116] and found O_2 consumption increased 2.6-fold.

In the Duck, arterial P_{O_2} remains unchanged while arterial P_{CO_2} even declines during exercise, indicating that the gas exchange system is capable of properly adjusting to the increased demand. The same may be true for the Hen, although only air sac gases, but no arterial blood gases, have been measured. The significant decline of mixed-venous P_{O_2} in the Duck, probably reflecting a decline in O_2 content, suggests that cardiac output increases less than O_2 uptake during exercise. This has also been reported for the walking Penguin (*Pygoscelis adeliae*)[122] and Duck.[118]

Table 3
RESPIRATION AND GAS EXCHANGE IN BIRDS RESTING
OR RUNNING ON A TREADMILL

	Domestic Hen[119-121,164]		Pekin Duck[116]	
	Rest	Exercise	Rest	Exercise
M_B (kg)	2.2		2.7	
Running speed ($m \cdot sec^{-1}$)	0	1.0	0	0.4
$\dot{M}_{O_2}$ ($mmol \cdot min^{-1}$)	1.70	4.91	—	—
$\dot{V}_I$ ($\ell \cdot min^{-1}$)	0.60	3.06	1.35	4.42
V_T ($m\ell$)	40	48	90	26
f_{resp} (min^{-1})	15	70	15	170
P_{O_2} (torr)				
Arterial	—	—	100	110
Mixed-venous	—	—	55	47
Mixed-expired	107	121	—	—
Clavicular air sac	95—101	110—112	—	—
Abdominal air sac	127	130	—	—
P_{CO_2} (torr)				
Arterial	—	—	25	19
Mixed-venous	—	—	29	25
Clavicular air sac	34	30	36	28
Abdominal air sac	17	15	—	—

Note: $\dot{V}_I$, total (inspired) ventilation. For other symbols, see Table 1.

3. Pharmacological Stimulation

Pulmonary gas exchange has recently been studied in the spontaneously breathing Duck when $\dot{M}_{O_2}$ was elevated by 2,4-dinitrophenol (DNP), a drug which increases metabolism by uncoupling oxidative phosphorylation.[86] With DNP, $\dot{M}_{O_2}$ could be made to increase up to sevenfold, and the pattern of response in the cardiorespiratory system showed striking similarities to those observed with natural hypermetabolism, like exercise.

In this preparation, a complete set of experimental variables could be measured which allowed a quantitative analysis of gas exchange. In particular, P_{O_2} and P_{CO_2} values were measured in arterial blood as well as in expired and clavicular air sac gases.

4. Cold

Exposure to a cold environment provides another tool to study respiration and gas exchange at stimulated metabolism. In the Pigeon, when ambient temperature is dropped from 22 to 2°C, both $\dot{M}_{O_2}$ and $\dot{V}_E$ increase about twofold and arterial blood gases remain nearly constant.[123] Cardiac output, on the other hand, increases less than $\dot{M}_{O_2}$, resulting in a significant drop in mixed-venous O_2 content and partial pressure. Unfortunately, respired gases were not measured. In parrots,[124] the Coot (*Fulica atra*),[125] and the Kittiwake (*Rissa tridactyla*),[126] cold exposure resulted in a reduction of the ventilatory requirement, i.e., of the ratio of total ventilation to O_2 uptake rate.

C. Hot Environment

Whereas during cold exposure the cardiorespiratory system has to adjust to the increased metabolic needs, it is for heat dissipation that ventilation increases during heat stress. Since birds do not possess sweat glands, panting is the main avenue for heat dissipation, aside from behavioral thermoregulation (see Chapter 6). The upper airways appear to be sites of

Table 4

RESPIRATION AND GAS EXCHANGE IN BIRDS EXPOSED TO MODERATE HEAT STRESS

	Pigeon[138]		Hen[135]		Duck[137]			Ostrich[93]	
T_A (°C)	—	—	20	37	20	25	35	20	40
T_B (°C)	41	43	42	43	41	41	42	39	43
f_{resp} (min^{-1})	28	549	15	174	10	38	260	6	50
		40[a]							
V_T (mℓ)	4	2.5	51	12[b]	80	66[b]	20	1400	1400
V_E ($\ell \cdot$ min^{-1})	0.11	0.10	0.79	2.09	0.80	2.50	5.20	8.4	70
V_D (mℓ)	1	1	8	8	13	13	13	400	400
V_P ($\ell \cdot$ min)	0.084	0.060	0.67	0.70	0.67	2.01	1.82	6.0	50.0
Pa_{CO_2} (torr)	25	27	26	25	30	29	28	—	—
pH_a	—	—	—	—	—	—	—	7.46	7.48

Note: Parabronchial ventilation, V_P, estimated as the difference between total ventilation, V_E, and dead space ventilation, assuming dead space volume, V_D, to equal tracheal volume. V_D not measured in Reference 137 but calculated from Hinds and Calder.[165] Other symbols as in Tables 1 and 2.

[a]   Slow component of compound ventilation.
[b]   Includes "flushing" breaths.

heat exchange[127-129] (cf. References 103 and 130), where a counter-current arrangement of blood and air flows provides an efficient system for heat dissipation.[131]

Typically, ventilation increases markedly in heat-stressed birds, but the effects of this increase on arterial blood gases differ between different bird species. While arterial P_{CO_2} has been found to fall to extremely low levels in a number of heat-stressed birds,[132-134] arterial P_{CO_2} and pH remained nearly constant in other species[134] (Domestic Fowl[135-137], Pigeon,[138] Rock Partridge [*Alectoris chukar*],[139] Ostrich [*Struthio camelus*],[20,93] Stork [*Sphenorhynchus alomii*][140]). Whether arterial homeostasis can be maintained depends largely on the extent of the heat stress. Bouverot et al.[137] have suggested that parabronchial hyperventilation, with ensuing hypocapnia, is prevented when ambient temperature is only moderately elevated, so there are no significant increases in body temperature. This "Phase I" panting thus indicates a functioning of the thermoregulatory system; it is characterized by a panting pattern of breathing, i.e., small tidal volume, V_T, and large respiratory frequency, f_{resp}. When, on the other hand, the heat stress is more severe, "Phase II" panting occurs, in which V_T increases, f_{resp} diminishes, and arterial hypocapnia occurs, indicating control systems regulating arterial blood gases are overridden by thermoregulatory controls.

Typical changes in respiration and gas exchange in birds exposed to moderate heat load (Phase I) are compiled in Table 4. It is evident that most birds maintained their body temperature (T_B), and arterial P_{CO_2} did not change significantly. Only in the study of Jones[93] did T_B increase significantly. Occurrence of hyperventilation in this study cannot be excluded from the arterial pH, pH_a, reported, since relatively constant pH_a may occur despite lowered Pa_{CO_2} as a result of lactic acid production in the stressed bird.

Several mechanisms may serve to prevent hyperventilation during thermal polypnea. First, changes in ventilatory pattern occur with decreased V_T and increased f_{resp} (= f) whereby the fraction of dead space ventilation increases and parabronchial ventilation is limited. However, as shown in Table 4, parabronchial ventilation increases in thermal stress and other mechanisms must be invoked to prevent arterial hypocapnia.

Bernstein and his colleagues[138,141,142] have demonstrated a compound pattern of ventilation in the pigeon comprising two components: a slow component (frequency similar to f_{resp} at rest) with large amplitude (similar to resting V_T); and a fast component (frequency close to natural resonant frequency of the animal; see Reference 143) with small amplitude (about one quarter of dead space volume). The authors suggest that the slow, deep component serves gas exchange, while the fast, shallow component ventilates the upper airways for heat exchange.

Alternations between small tidal volumes, smaller than V_D, and larger "flushing" breaths have been observed in the panting Flamingo (*Phoenicopterus ruber*).[144-146] In reviewing the literature, these authors suggest that this type of switching between deep (gas exchange) breaths and shallow (heat exchange) breaths occurred also in the Fowl of Brackenbury et al.[135] and, at 25°C, the Duck of Bouverot et al.[137]

In mammals, gas exchange can be maintained with tidal volumes below anatomic dead space volume and with respiratory frequency at or above 1200 min^{-1}. The mechanism for gas transport under these conditions of high frequency ventilation (HFV) is not exactly known, but convective axial dispersion in the conducting airways is responsible[147,148] (cf. Reference 149). Hastings and Powell[150] and Banzett and Lehr[151] have shown that HFV can maintain gas exchange in the Duck. In the study of Hastings and Powell,[150] f_{resp} had to be greater than that reported for heat-stressed Ducks (Table 4). Thus it is not clear whether similar mechanisms provide gas transport during panting and during HFV.

A second potential mechanism to prevent hyperventilation with thermal polypnea is an increased ventilatory shunt past the parabronchial lung. This was proposed by Jones[93] for the Ostrich in which nondead space ventilation increases markedly (Table 4). Zeuthen[18] has proposed an increase in parabronchial smooth muscle tone whereby parabronchial airflow resistance would be increased, as would be the amount of air shunted past the parabronchi. Molony et al.[152] found the resistance of the medioventral secondary bronchi to increase with decreasing CO_2 in the ventilating gas, but parabronchial air flow resistance remained largely unaffected. These authors suggested that during panting, CO_2 at the ventrobronchi may decrease, resulting in an increased airflow resistance through the parabronchial lung.

D. Altitude

At extreme altitude, various factors, such as low O_2 partial pressure, cold, low air density, and cosmic radiation may limit survival. The highest altitude which acclimatized man has been able to reach without supplemental oxygen is that of Mt. Everest, 8848 m,[153] but his capacity to exercise under these conditions is extremely limited.[154] Diffusion across the alveolar-capillary barrier has been identified as a major limiting factor in gas transfer under these conditions.[155,156]

There are several reports on birds flying at altitudes that man has not reached without supplemental O_2.[157-160] Studies in which birds were acutely exposed to low levels of O_2 suggest that at least birds with good power of flight can tolerate altitudes and low levels of O_2 that would incapacitate man.[66] The most amazing avian performance at altitude is that of the Bar-Headed Goose (*Anser indicus*), which has been reported to fly without acclimatization across the summit of Mt. Everest.[157] In the laboratory, this bird at rest tolerated inspired P_{O_2} as low as 23 torr, corresponding to an altitude of 11,600 m.[66] These authors measured blood gases and found Pa_{O_2} to be very close to inspired P_{O_2}, and Pa_{CO_2} to be below 8 torr. This suggests very efficient gas exchange in this animal. Calculations suggest that the inherent efficiency of the parabronchial gas exchange system is important in the high altitude tolerance of birds, but that other factors must contribute. One such factor may be the reported lack of hypocapnic vasoconstriction in brain vessels[161] which may allow ventilation to rise to higher levels than in mammals without ill effects of the ensuing hypocapnia, particularly for brain perfusion and O_2 supply.

The exquisite tolerance of hypoxia that some birds exhibit could, at least in part, be caused by the peculiarly high gas exchange efficiency of the avian lung. It might, in fact, be expected that this advantage in efficiency that birds have over mammals is particularly prominent in the stressful situation of deep hypoxia.

Scheid[152a] has tried to estimate this advantage. He has used measurements and estimates of man at the altitude of Mt. Everest[153,154] and calculated blood gas for this man on the assumption that his alveolar lung was replaced by a parabronchial lung. The calculations show that this man could ascend to about 780 m higher altitude for the same arterial blood gases. This constitutes a significant advantage provided by the cross-current system. However, birds have been observed to fly at substantially higher altitude so that factors other than the high lung efficiency must be invoked. These factors may reside in tissue gas exchange or in the reactivity of capillaries to hypoxia and hypocapnia, but further research is needed to help answer this question.

REFERENCES

1. **Piiper, J. and Scheid, P.,** Blood-gas equilibration in lungs, in *Pulmonary Gas Exchange,* Vol. 1, West, J. B., Ed., Academic Press, London, 1980, 131.
2. **Piiper, J., Drees, F., and Scheid, P.,** Gas exchange in the domestic fowl during spontaneous breathing and artificial ventilation, *Respir. Physiol.,* 9, 234, 1970.
3. **Scheid, P. and Piiper, J.,** Analysis of gas exchange in the avian lung: theory and experiments in the domestic fowl, *Respir. Physiol.,* 9, 246, 1970.
4. **Piiper, J. and Scheid, P.,** Gas transport efficacy of gills, lungs and skin: theory and experimental data, *Respir. Physiol.,* 23, 209, 1975.
5. **Scheid, P. and Piiper, J.,** Blood-gas equilibrium of carbon dioxide in lungs, A review, *Respir. Physiol.,* 39, 1, 1980.
6. **Akester, A. R.,** The comparative anatomy of the respiratory pathways in the domestic fowl (*Gallus domesticus*), pigeon (*Columba livia*), and domestic duck (*Anas platyrhynchos*), *J. Anat.,* 94, 487, 1960.
7. **Duncker, H.-R.,** The lung air sac system of birds, *Ergebn. Anat. Entwicklungsgesch.,* 45/6, 1, 1971.
8. **Duncker, H.-R.,** Structure of avian lungs, *Respir. Physiol.,* 14, 44, 1972.
9. **Duncker, H.-R.,** Structure of the avian respiratory tract, *Respir. Physiol.,* 22, 1, 1974.
10. **King, A. S.,** Structural and functional aspects of the avian lungs and air sacs, *Int. Rev. Gen. Exp. Zool.,* 2, 171, 1966.
11. **King, A. S.,** Aves, respiratory system, in *The Anatomy of the Domestic Animals,* Vol. 2, 5th ed., Getty, R., Ed., Saunders, Philadelphia, 1975, 1883.
12. **King, A. S. and Molony, V.,** The anatomy of respiration, in *Physiology and Biochemistry of the Domestic Fowl,* Vol. 1, Bell, D. K. and Freeman, B. M., Eds., Academic Press, London, 1971, 93.
13. **Magnussen, H., Willmer, H., and Scheid, P.,** Gas exchange in air sacs: contribution to respiratory gas exchange in ducks, *Respir. Physiol.,* 26, 129, 1976.
14. **King, A. S. and Cowie, A. F.,** The functional anatomy of the bronchial muscle of the bird, *J. Anat.,* 105, 323, 1969.
15. **Macklem, P. T., Bouverot, P., and Scheid, P.,** Measurement of the distensibility of the parabronchi in duck lung, *Respir. Physiol.,* 38, 23, 1979.
16. **Fedde, M. R., Burger, R. E., and Kitchell, R. L.,** Anatomic and electromyographic studies of the costopulmonary muscles in the cock, *Poult. Sci.,* 43, 1177, 1964.
17. **Vos, H. F.,** Über die Wege der Atemluft in der Entenlunge, *Z. Vergl. Physiol.,* 21, 552, 1935.
18. **Zeuthen, E.,** The ventilation of the respiratory tract in birds, *K. Dan. Vidensk. Selsk. Biol. Medd.,* 17, 1, 1942.
19. **Shepard, R. H., Sladen, B. K., Peterson, N., and Enns, T.,** Path taken by gases through the respiratory system of the chicken, *J. Appl. Physiol.,* 14, 733, 1959.
20. **Schmidt-Nielsen, K., Kanwisher, J., Lasieski, R. C., Cohn, J. E., and Bretz, W. L.,** Temperature regulation and respiration in the ostrich, *Condor,* 71, 341, 1969.
21. **Bouverot, P. and Dejours, P.,** Pathway of respired gas in the air sacs-lung apparatus of fowl and ducks, *Respir. Physiol.,* 13, 330, 1971.
22. **Bretz, W. L. and Schmidt-Nielsen, K.,** Bird respiration: flow patterns in the duck lung, *J. Exp. Biol.,* 54, 103, 1971.

23. **Scheid, P., Slama, H., and Willmer, H.,** Volume and ventilation of air sacs in ducks studied by inert gas wash-out, *Respir. Physiol.,* 21, 19, 1974.
24. **Torre-Bueno, J. R., Geiser, J., and Scheid, P.,** Incomplete gas mixing in air sacs of the duck, *Respir. Physiol.,* 42, 109, 1980.
25. **Biggs, P. M. and King, A. S.,** A new experimental approach to the problem of the air pathway within the avian lung, *J. Physiol.,* 138, 282, 1957.
26. **King, J. R. and Farner, D. S.,** Terrestrial animals in humid heat: birds, in *Handbook of Physiology,* Section 4, *Adaptation to the Environment,* Dill, D. B., Adolph, E. F., and Wilber, C. G., Eds., American Physiological Society, Washington, D.C., 1964, 603.
27. **Scheid, P.,** Mechanisms of gas exchange in bird lungs, *Rev. Physiol. Biochem. Pharmacol.,* 86, 137, 1979.
28. **Dotterweich, H.,** Die Bahnhofstaube und die Frage nach dem Weg der Atemluft, *Zool. Anz.,* 90, 259, 1930.
29. **Dotterweich, H.,** Versuch über den Weg der Atemluft in der Vogellunge, *Z. Vergl. Physiol.,* 11, 271, 1930.
30. **Walter, W. G.,** Beiträge zur Frage über den Weg der Luft in den Atmungsorganen der Vögel, *Arch. Neerl. Physiol.,* 19, 529, 1934.
31. **Graham, J. D. P.,** The air stream in the lung of the fowl, *J. Physiol.,* 97, 133, 1939.
32. **Hazelhoff, E. H.,** Bouw en functie van de vogellong, *Versl. Gewone Vergad. Afd. Natuurk. Kon. Ned. Akad. Wet.,* 52, 391, 1943; Structure and function of the lung of birds, *Poultry Sci.,* 30, 3, 1951.
33. **Dotterweich, H.,** Ein weiterer Beitrag zur Atmungsphysiologie der Vögel, *Z. Vergl. Physiol.,* 18, 803, 1933.
34. **Makowski, J.,** Beitrag zur Klärung des Atmungsmechanismus der Vögel, *Pflügers Arch.,* 240, 407, 1938.
35. **Scharnke, H.,** Experimentelle Beiträge zur Kenntnis der Vogelatmung, *Z. Vergl. Physiol.,* 25, 548, 1938.
36. **Cohn, J. E. and Shannon, R.,** Respiration in unanesthetized geese, *Respir. Physiol.,* 5, 259, 1968.
37. **Dotterweich, H.,** Die Atmung der Vögel, *Z. Vergl. Physiol.,* 23, 744, 1936.
38. **James, A. E., Hutchins, G., Bush, M., Natarajan, T. K., and Burns, B.,** How birds breathe: correlation of radiographic with anatomical and pathological studies, *J. Am. Vet. Radiol. Soc.,* 17, 77, 1976.
39. **Burns, B., James, A. E., Hutchins, G., Novak, G., and Price, R. R.,** Ventilatory [133]xenon distribution studies in the duck (*Anas platyrhynchos*), in *Respiratory Function in Birds, Adult and Embryonic,* Piiper, J., Ed., Springer, Berlin, 1978, 129.
40. **Bretz, W. L. and Schmidt-Nielsen, K.,** Patterns of air flow in the duck lung, *Fed. Proc.,* 29, 662, 1970.
41. **Scheid, P. and Piiper, J.,** Direkte Messung der Strömungsrichtung der Atemluft in der Entenlunge, *Pflügers Arch.,* 319, R59, 1970.
42. **Scheid, P. and Piiper, J.,** Direct measurement of the pathway of respired gas in duck lungs, *Respir. Physiol.,* 11, 308, 1971.
43. **Brackenbury, J. H.,** Airflow dynamics in the avian lung as determined by direct and indirect methods, *Respir. Physiol.,* 13, 319, 1971.
44. **Bethe, A.,** Atmung: Allgemeines und Vergleichendes, in *Handbuch der normalen und pathologischen Physiologie,* Vol. 2, Bethe, A., Bergmann, G. v., Embden, G., and Ellinger, A., Eds., Springer, Berlin, 1925, 1.
45. **Bretz, W. L. and Schmidt-Nielsen, K.,** The movement of gas in the respiratory system of the duck, *J. Exp. Biol.,* 56, 57, 1972.
46. **Portier, P.,** Sur le rôle physiologique des sacs aériens des oiseaux, *Compt. Rend. Soc. Biol.,* 99, 1327, 1928.
47. **Scheid, P. and Piiper, J.,** Cross-current gas exchange in avian lungs: effects of reversed parabronchial air flow in ducks, *Respir. Physiol.,* 16, 304, 1972.
48. **Powell, F. L., Geiser, J., Gratz, R. K., and Scheid, P.,** Airflow in the avian respiratory tract: variations of O_2 and CO_2 concentrations in the bronchi of the duck, *Respir. Physiol.,* 44, 195, 1981.
49. **Brandes, G.,** Beobachtungen und Reflexionen über die Atmung der Vögel, *Pflügers Arch.,* 203, 492, 1924.
50. **King, A. S. and Payne, D. C.,** Does the air circulate in the avian lung?, *Anat. Rec.,* 136, 223, 1960.
51. **Brackenbury, J. H.,** Lung-air sac anatomy and respiratory pressures in the bird, *J. Exp. Biol.,* 57, 543, 1972.
52. **Brackenbury, J. H.,** Corrections to the Hazelhoff model of airflow in the avian lung, *Respir. Physiol.,* 36, 143, 1979.
53. **Brackenbury, J. H.,** Physical determinants of air flow pattern within the avian lung, *Respir. Physiol.,* 15, 384, 1972.
54. **Molony, V., Graf, W., and Scheid, P.,** Effects of CO_2 on pulmonary air flow resistance in the duck, *Respir. Physiol.,* 26, 333, 1976.
55. **Schmidt-Nielsen, K.,** How birds breathe, *Sci. Am.,* 225(6), 72, 1971.

56. **Piiper, J. and Scheid, P.,** Gas exchange in avian lungs: models and experimental evidence, in *Comparative Physiology,* Bolis, L., Schmidt-Nielsen, K., and Maddrell, S. H. P., Eds., North-Holland, Amsterdam, 1973, 161.

57. **Scheid, P., Worth, H., Holle, J. P., and Meyer, M.,** Effects of oscillating and intermittent ventilatory flow on efficacy of pulmonary O_2 transfer in the duck, *Respir. Physiol.,* 31, 251, 1977.

58. **Scheid, P.,** Estimation of effective parabronchial gas volume during intermittent ventilatory flow: theory and application in the duck, *Respir. Physiol.,* 32, 1, 1978.

59. **Scheid, P., Slama, H., Gatz, R. N., and Fedde, M. R.,** Intrapulmonary CO_2 receptors in the duck. III. Functional localization, *Respir. Physiol.,* 22, 123, 1974.

60. **Fedde, M. R.,** Respiration, in *Avian Physiology,* 3rd ed., Sturkie, P. D., Ed., Springer, Berlin, 1976, 122.

61. **Bouverot, P.,** Control of breathing in birds as compared with mammals, *Physiol. Rev.,* 58, 604, 1978.

62. **Piiper, J.,** Origin of carbon dioxide in caudal air sacs of birds, in *Respiratory Function in Birds, Adult and Embryonic,* Piiper, J., Ed., Springer, Berlin, 1978, 148.

63. **Sturkie, P. D.,** Blood: physical characteristics, formed elements, hemoglobin and coagulation, in *Avian Physiology,* Sturkie, P. D., Ed., Springer, New York, 1976, 54.

64. **Lutz, P. L., Longmuir, I. S., and Schmidt-Nielsen, K.,** Oxygen affinity of bird blood, *Respir. Physiol.,* 20, 325, 1974.

65. **Lapennas, G. N. and Reeves, R. B.,** Oxygen affinity of blood of adult domestic chicken and red jungle fowl, *Respir. Physiol.,* 52, 27, 1983.

66. **Black, C. P. and Tenney, S. M.,** Oxygen transport during progressive hypoxia in high altitude and sea-level water-fowl, *Respir. Physiol.,* 39, 217, 1980.

67. **Johnson, L. F. and Tate, M. E.,** Structure of 'phytic acid', *Canad. J. Chem.,* 47, 63, 1969.

68. **Bartlett, G. R.,** Pattern of phosphate compounds in red blood cells of man and animals, in *Red Cell Metabolism and Function,* Brewer, G. J., Ed., Plenum, New York, 1970, 245.

69. **Weingarten, J. P., Rollema, H. S., Bauer, C., and Scheid, P.,** Effects of inositol hexaphosphate on the Bohr effect induced by CO_2 and fixed acid in chicken hemoglobin, *Pflügers Arch.,* 377, 135, 1978.

70. **Wells, R. M. G.,** The oxygen affinity of chicken hemoglobin in whole blood and erythrocyte suspensions, *Respir. Physiol.,* 27, 21, 1976.

71. **Meyer, M., Holle, J. P., and Scheid, P.,** Bohr effect induced by CO_2 and fixed acid at various levels of O_2 saturation in duck blood, *Pflügers Arch.,* 376, 237, 1978.

72. **Tazawa, H. and Piiper, J.,** Carbon dioxide dissociation and buffering in chicken blood during development, *Respir. Physiol.,* 57, 123, 1984.

73. **Scheipers, G., Kawashiro, T, and Scheid, P.,** Oxygen and carbon dioxide dissociation of duck blood, *Respir. Physiol.,* 24, 1, 1975.

74. **Kawashiro, T. and Scheid, P.,** Arterial blood gases in undisturbed resting birds: measurements in chicken and duck, *Respir. Physiol.,* 23, 337, 1975.

75. **Piiper, J. and Scheid, P.,** Physical principles of respiratory gas exchange in fish gills, in *Gills,* Houlihan, D. F., Rankin, J. C., and Shuttleworth, T. J., Eds., Cambridge University Press, Cambridge, 1982, 45.

76. **Piiper, J. and Scheid, P.,** Comparative physiology of respiration: functional analysis of gas exchange organs in vertebrates, in *International Review of Physiology, Series II, Respiratory Physiology II,* Vol. 14, Widdicombe, J. G., Ed., University Park Press, Baltimore, 1977, 219.

77. **Scheid, P.,** Analysis of gas exchange between air capillaries and blood capillaries in avian lungs, *Respir. Physiol.,* 32, 27, 1978.

78. **Meyer, M., Worth, H., and Scheid, P.,** Gas-blood CO_2 equilibration in parabronchial lungs of birds, *J. Appl. Physiol.,* 41, 302, 1976.

79. **Davies, D. G. and Dutton, R. E.,** Gas-blood P_{CO_2} gradients during avian gas exchange, *J. Appl. Physiol.,* 39, 405, 1975.

80. **Piiper, J., Dejours, P., Haab, P., and Rahn, H.,** Concepts and basic quantities in gas exchange physiology, *Respir. Physiol.,* 13, 292, 1971.

81. **Crank, W. D. and Gallagher, R. R.,** Theory of gas exchange in the avian parabronchus, *Respir. Physiol.,* 35, 9, 1978.

82. **Akester, A. R.,** The blood vascular system, in *Physiology and Biochemistry of the Domestic Fowl,* Vol. 2, Bell, D. J. and Freeman, B. M., Eds., Academic Press, London, 1971, 783.

83. **Abdalla, M. A. and King, A. S.,** The functional anatomy of the pulmonary circulation of the domestic fowl, *Respir. Physiol.,* 23, 267, 1975.

84. **Burger, R. E., Meyer, M., Graf, W., and Scheid, P.,** Gas exchange in the parabronchial lung of birds: experiments in unidirectionally ventilated ducks, *Respir. Physiol.,* 36, 19, 1979.

85. **Scheid, P., Gratz, R. K., Powell, F. L., and Fedde, M. R.,** Ventilatory response to CO_2 in birds. II. Contribution by intrapulmonary CO_2 receptors, *Respir. Physiol.,* 35, 361, 1978.

86. **Geiser, J., Gratz, R. K., Hiramoto, T., and Scheid, P.,** Effects of increasing metabolism by 2,4-dinitrophenol on respiration and pulmonary gas exchange in the duck, *Resp. Physiol.,* 57, 1, 1984.

87. **Powell, F. L. and Wagner, P. D.,** Measurement of continuous distributions of ventilation-perfusion in non-alveolar lungs, *Respir. Physiol.,* 48, 219, 1982.

88. **Powell, F. L. and Wagner, P. D.,** Ventilation-perfusion inequality in avian lungs, *Respir. Physiol.,* 48, 233, 1982.

89. **Powell, F. L. and Scheid, P.,** Physiology of gas exchange in the avian respiratory system, in *Form and Function in Birds,* Vol. 4, King, A. S., Ed., Academic Press, London, in press.

90. **Holle, J. P., Heisler, N., and Scheid, P.,** Blood flow distribution in the duck lung and its control by respiratory gases, *Am. J. Physiol.,* 234, R146, 1978.

91. **Parry, K. and Yates, M. S.,** Observations on the avian pulmonary and bronchial circulation using labelled microspheres, *J. Anat. (London),* 127, 199, 1978.

92. **Parry, K. and Yates, M. S.,** Observations on the avian pulmonary and bronchial circulation using labelled microspheres, *Respir. Physiol.,* 38, 131, 1979.

93. **Jones, J. H.,** Pulmonary blood flow distribution in panting ostriches, *J. Appl. Physiol.: Respirat. Environ. Exercise Physiol.,* 53, 1411, 1982.

94. **Wagner, P. D. and West, J. B.,** Ventilation-perfusion relationships, in *Pulmonary Gas Exchange,* Vol. I, West, J. B., Ed., Academic Press, San Francisco, 1980, 219.

95. **Jammes, Y. and Bouverot, P.,** Direct P_{CO_2} measurements in the dorsobronchial gas of awake Peking ducks: evidence for a physiological role of the neopulmo in respiratory gas exchanges, *Comp. Biochem. Physiol.,* 52A, 635, 1975.

96. **Abdalla, M. A., Maina, J. N., King, A. S., King, D. Z., and Henry, J.,** Morphometrics of the avian lung. I. The domestic fowl (*Gallus gallus variant domesticus*), *Respir. Physiol.,* 47, 267, 1982.

97. **Maina, J. N. and King, A. S.,** Morphometrics of the avian lung. 2. The wild mallard (*Anas platyrhynchos*) and graylag goose (*Anser anser*), *Respir. Physiol.,* 50, 299, 1982.

98. **Maina, J. N.,** Morphometrics of the avian lung. 3. The structural design of the passerine lung, *Respir. Physiol.,* 55, 291, 1984.

99. **Crapo, J. D. and Crapo, R. O.,** Comparison of total lung diffusion capacity and the membrane component of diffusion capacity as determined by physiologic and morphometric techniques, *Respir. Physiol.,* 51, 183, 1983.

100. **Scheid, P. and Slama, H.,** Remote-controlled device for sampling arterial blood in unrestrained animals, *Pflügers Arch.,* 356, 373, 1975.

101. **Lasiewski, R. C. and Dawson, W. R.,** A re-examination of the relation between standard metabolic rate and body weight in birds, *Condor,* 69, 13, 1967.

102. **Lasiewski, R. C. and Calder, W. A.,** A preliminary allometric analysis of respiratory variables in resting birds, *Respir. Physiol.,* 11, 152, 1971.

103. **Lasiewski, R. C.,** Respiratory function in birds, in *Avian Biology,* Vol. 2, Farner, D. S. and King, J. R., Eds., Academic Press, New York, 1972, 287.

104. **King, A. S. and King, D. Z.,** Avian morphology: general principles, in *Form and Function in Birds,* Vol. 1, King, A. S. and McLelland, J., Eds., Academic Press, London, 1979, 1.

105. **Powell, F. L.,** in *Physiology and Behaviour of the Pigeon,* Abs, M., Ed., Academic Press, New York, 1983, 73.

106. **Berger, M. and Hart, J. S.,** Physiology and energetics of flight, in *Avian Biology,* Vol. 4, Farner, D. S. and King, J. R., Eds., Academic Press, New York, 1974, 415.

107. **Seeherman, H. J., Taylor, C. R., Maloiy, G. M. O., and Armstrong, R. B.,** Design of the mammalian respiratory system, II. Measuring maximum aerobic capacity, *Respir. Physiol.,* 44, 11, 1981.

108. **Berger, M.,** Oxygen consumption and power of hovering hummingbirds at varying barometric and oxygen pressures, *Naturwissenschaften,* 61, 407, 1974.

109. **Berger, M.,** Ventilation in the humming birds *Colibri coruscans* during altitude hovering, in *Respiratory Function in Birds, Adult and Embryonic,* Piiper, J., Ed., Springer, Berlin, 1978, 85.

110. **Berger, M., Hart, J. S., and Roy, O. Z.,** Respiration, oxygen consumption and heart rate in some birds during rest and flight, *Z. Vgl. Physiol.,* 66, 201, 1970.

111. **Lasiewski, R. C.,** Oxygen consumption of torpid, resting, active and flying hummingbirds, *Physiol. Zool.,* 36, 122, 1963.

112. **Butler, P. J. and Woakes, A. J.,** Heart rate, respiratory frequency and wing beat frequency of free flying Barnacle Geese *Branta leucopsis.*, *J. Exp. Biol.,* 82, 213, 1980.

113. **Tucker, V. A.,** Oxygen consumption of a flying bird, *Science,* 154, 150, 1966.

114. **Torre-Bueno, J. R.,** Respiration during flight in birds, in *Respiratory Function in Birds, Adult and Embryonic,* Piiper, J., Ed., Springer, Berlin, 1978, 89.

115. **Butler, P. J., West, N. H., and Jones, D. R.,** Respiratory and cardiovascular response of the pigeon to sustained, level flight in a wind-tunnel, *J. Exp. Biol.,* 71, 7, 1977.

116. **Kiley, J. P., Kuhlmann, W. D., and Fedde, M. R.,** Respiratory and cardiovascular responses to exercise in the duck, *J. Appl. Physiol.: Respirat. Environ. Exercise Physiol.,* 47, 827, 1979.

117. **Grubb, B. R.,** Cardiac output and stroke volume in exercising ducks and pigeons, *J. Appl. Physiol.: Respirat. Environ. Exercise Physiol.,* 53, 207, 1982.

118. **Bech, C. and Nomoto, S.,** Cardiovascular changes associated with treadmill running in the Peking duck, *J. Exp. Biol.,* 97, 345, 1982.

119. **Brackenbury, J. H., Avery, P., and Gleeson, M.,** Respiration in exercising fowl. I. Oxygen consumption, respiratory rate and respired gases, *J. Exp. Biol.,* 93, 317, 1981.

120. **Brackenbury, J. H., Gleeson, M., and Avery, P.,** Effects of sustained running exercise on lung air-sac gas composition and respiratory pattern in domestic fowl, *Comp. Biochem. Physiol.,* 69A, 449, 1981.

121. **Brackenbury, J. H. and Avery, P.,** Energy consumption and ventilatory mechanisms in the exercising fowl, *Comp. Biochem. Physiol.,* 66A, 439, 1980.

122. **Millard, R. W., Johansen, K., and Milsom, W. K.,** Radiotelemetry of cardiovascular responses to exercise and during diving in penguins, *Comp. Biochem. Physiol.,* 46A, 227, 1973.

123. **Bouverot, P., Hildwein, G., and Oulhen, P.,** Ventilatory and circulatory O_2 convection at 4000 m in pigeon at neutral or cold temperature, *Respir. Physiol.,* 28, 371, 1976.

124. **Bucher, T. L.,** Oxygen consumption, ventilation and respiratory heat loss in a parrot, *Bolborhynchus lineola,* in relation to ambient temperature, *J. Comp. Physiol.,* 142, 479, 1981.

125. **Brent, R., Pedersen, P. F., Bech, C., and Johansen, K.,** Lung ventilation and temperature regulation in the European coot *Fulica atra, Physiol. Zool.,* 57, 19, 1984.

126. **Brent, R., Rasmussen, J. G., Bech, C., and Martini, S.,** Temperature dependence of ventilation and O_2-extraction in the Kittiwake (*Rissa tridactyla*), *Experientia,* 39, 1092, 1983.

127. **Schmidt-Nielsen, K., Hainsworth, F. R., and Murrish, D. E.,** Counter-current heat exchange in the respiratory passages: effect on water and heat balance, *Respir. Physiol.,* 9, 263, 1970.

128. **Murrish, D. E.,** Respiratory heat and water exchange in penguins, *Respir. Physiol.,* 19, 262, 1973.

129. **Menuam, B. and Richards, S. A.,** Observations on the sites of respiratory evaporation in the fowl during thermal panting, *Respir. Physiol.,* 25, 39, 1975.

130. **Schmidt-Nielsen, K.,** *How Animals Work,* Cambridge University Press, Cambridge, 1972.

131. **Jackson, D. C. and Schmidt-Nielsen, K.,** Countercurrent heat heat exchange in the respiratory passages, *Proc. Natl. Acad. Sci. U.S.A.,* 51, 1192, 1964.

132. **Linsley, J. G. and Burger, R. E.,** Respiratory and cardiovascular responses in the hyperthermic domestic cock, *Poult. Sci.,* 43, 291, 1964.

133. **Calder, W. A. and Schmidt-Nielsen, K.,** Evaporative cooling and respiratory alkalosis in the pigeon, *Proc. Natl. Acad. Sci. U.S.A.,* 55, 750, 1966.

134. **Calder, W. A. and Schmidt-Nielsen, K.,** Panting and blood carbon dioxide in birds, *Am. J. Physiol.,* 215, 477, 1968.

135. **Brackenbury, J. H., Avery, P., and Gleeson, M.,** Air sac gases and ventilation during panting in fowl, *Gallus gallus, J. Exp. Biol.,* 90, 343, 1981.

136. **Marder, J., Arad, Z., and Gafni, M.,** The effect of high ambient temperature on acid-base balance of panting Bedouin fowl (*Gallus domesticus*), *Physiol. Zool.,* 47, 180, 1974.

137. **Bouverot, P., Hildwein, G., and Le Goff, D.,** Evaporative water loss, respiratory pattern, gas exchange and acid-base balance during thermal panting in Pekin ducks exposed to moderate heat, *Respir. Physiol.,* 21, 255, 1974.

138. **Bernstein, M. H. and Samaniego, F. C.,** Ventilation and acid-base status during thermal panting in pigeons (*Columba livia*), *Physiol. Zool.,* 54, 308, 1981.

139. **Krausz, S., Bernstein, R., and Marder, J.,** The acid base balance of the rock partridge (*Alectoris chukar*) exposed to high ambient temperatures, *Comp. Biochem. Physiol.,* 57A, 245, 1977.

140. **Marder, J. and Arad, Z.,** The acid base balance of Abdim's stork (*Sphenorhynchus abdimii*) during thermal panting, *Comp. Biochem. Physiol.,* 51A, 887, 1975.

141. **Ramirez, J. M. and Bernstein, M. H.,** Compound ventilation during thermal panting in pigeons: a possible mechanism for minimizing hypocapnic alkalosis, *Fed. Proc.,* 35, 2562, 1976.

142. **Hudson, D. M. and Bernstein, M. H.,** Respiratory ventilation during steady-state flight in the white-necked raven, *Corvus cryptoleucus, Fed. Proc.,* 37, 472, 1978.

143. **Crawford, E. C. Jr. and Kampe, G.,** Resonant panting in pigeons, *Comp. Biochem. Physiol.,* 40A, 549, 1971.

144. **Bech, C. and Johansen, K.,** Blood-flow changes in the duck during thermal panting, *Acta Physiol. Scand.,* 110, 351, 1980.

145. **Bech, C., Johansen, K., and Maloiy, G. M. O.,** Ventilation and expired gas composition in the flamingo, *Phoenicopterus ruber,* during normal respiration and panting, *Physiol. Zool.,* 52, 313, 1979.

146. **Johansen, K. and Bech, C.,** Breathing and thermoregulation in birds, in *Thermal Physiology,* Hales, J. R. S., Ed., Raven Press, N.Y., 1984, 341.

147. **Knopp, T. J., Kaethner, T., Meyer, M., Rehder, K., and Scheid, P.,** Gas mixing in the airways of dog lungs during high-frequency ventilation, *J. Appl. Physiol.: Respirat. Environ. Exercise Physiol.,* 55, 1141, 1983.

148. **Kaethner, T., Kohl, J., and Scheid, P.,** Gas concentration profiles along the airways of dog lungs during high frequency ventilation, *J. Appl. Physiol.: Respirat. Environ. Exercise Physiol.,* 56, 1491, 1984.

149. **Piiper, J. and Scheid, P.,** Diffusion and convection in intrapulmonary gas mixing, in *Handbook of Physiology Respiration,* Vol. 3: *Gas Exchange,* Farhi, L. E., Ed., American Physiological Society, Bethesda, 1985, in press.

150. **Hastings, R. H. and Powell, F. L.,** CO_2 elimination in ducks is maintained by high frequency ventilation with tidal volume less than dead space, *Fed. Proc.,* 41, 1096, 1982.

151. **Banzett, R. B. and Lehr, J. L.,** Gas exchange during high-frequency ventilation of the chicken, *J. Appl. Physiol.: Respirat. Environ. Exercise Physiol.,* 53, 1418, 1982.

152. **Molony, V., Graf, W., and Scheid, P.,** Effects of CO_2 on pulmonary air flow resistance in the duck, *Respir. Physiol.,* 26, 333, 1976.

152a. **Scheid, P.,** Significance of lung structure for performance at high altitude, in *Acta XVIII Congr. Int. Ornithologici,* Vol. III, Ilyicher, V. D. and Gavrilov, V. M., Eds., Nauka, Moscow, 1985, 976.

153. **Dejours, P.,** Mount Everest and beyond: breating air, in *A Companion to Animal Physiology,* Taylor, C. R., Johansen, K., and Bolis, L., Eds., Cambridge University Press, Cambridge, 1982, 17.

154. **West, J. B.,** Climbing Mt. Everest without oxygen: an analysis of maximal exercise during extreme hypoxia, *Respir. Physiol.,* 52, 265, 1983.

155. **West, J. B. and Wagner, P. D.,** Predicted gas exchange on the summit of Mt. Everest, *Respir. Physiol.,* 42, 1, 1980.

156. **Piiper, J. and Scheid, P.,** Model for capillary-alveolar equilibration with special reference to O_2 uptake in hypoxia, *Respir. Physiol.,* 46, 193, 1981.

157. **Hunt, J.,** *The Conquest of Everest,* Dutton, New York, 1954.

158. **Manville, R. H.,** Altitude record for Mallard, *Wilson Bull.,* 75, 92, 1963.

159. **Swan, L. W.,** Goose of the Himalayas, *Nat. Hist.,* 79, 68, 1970.

160. **Luft, U. C.,** Aviation physiology — the effects of altitude, in *Handbook of Physiology,* Fenn, W. O. and Rahn, H., Eds., William & Wilkins, Baltimore, 1965.

161. **Grubb, B. R., Mills, C. D., Colacino, J. M., and Schmidt-Nielsen, K.,** Effect of arterial carbon dioxide on cerebral blood flow in ducks, *Am. J. Physiol.,* 232, H596, 1977.

162. **Bouverot, P., Douguet, D., and Sébert, P.,** Role of the arterial chemoreceptors in ventilatory and circulatory adjustments to hypoxia in awake Pekin ducks, *J. Comp. Physiol.,* 133, 177, 1979.

163. **Jones, D. R. and Holeton, G. F.,** Cardiovascular and respiratory responses of ducks to progressive hypocapnic hypoxia, *J. Exp. Biol.,* 56, 657, 1972.

164. **Brackenbury, J. H., Gleeson, M., and Avery, P.,** Respiration in exercising fowl. III. Ventilation, *J. Exp. Biol.,* 96, 315, 1982.

165. **Hinds, D. S. and Calder, W. A.,** Tracheal deadspace in the respiration of birds, *Evolution,* 25, 429, 1971.

Chapter 5

TEMPERATURE CONTROL

G. M. Barnas and W. Rautenberg

TABLE OF CONTENTS

I. INTRODUCTION

The evolution of homeothermia in birds was not accompanied by development of specific effector organs able to correct deviations of body temperature under cold or heat conditions. In defense against a cold load, the internal heat production of a bird is increased by shivering thermogenesis caused by tremor of skeletal muscles; there is no evidence of brown adipose tissue in birds, which produces nonshivering thermogenesis in many mammalian species. The increase in heat dissipation in response to a heat load is controlled by changes in respiratory evaporation in avian species; regulation of cutaneous evaporation by secretion of sweat glands, as in the case of mammals, is not applicable in birds. This means that birds regulate their body temperature by using effector organs or organ systems which were primarily developed in their ectothermic ancestors for regulating other controlled variables, e.g., muscle contraction, blood gases, and acid-base balance. This incorporation of one or more feedback control systems to serve temperature regulation results in interaction, and sometimes competition, of the involved control functions and may unavoidably influence the adjustments made in controlled variables.

In this chapter we report on results which have dealt with the interaction between the respiratory- and temperature-control systems in birds and the influence on the controlled variables involved. Many investigations have been made to characterize the interaction between these systems during heat stress, when birds must force their respiration to dissipate heat by evaporation. However, relatively few authors have studied the two systems and their variables in response to a cold environment.

II. RESPIRATION DURING HYPERTHERMIA

A. Modes of Heat Loss

Birds, being homeothermic, must dissipate a quantity of heat equivalent to their metabolic heat production by losing heat to their environment, otherwise body temperature will begin to increase. The most important mode of heat loss at high ambient temperatures is that of evaporation of water, since other routes — conduction convection, and radiation — are directly related to the temperature gradient between the environment and the body surface. Indeed, at ambient temperature (T_a) near that of the body temperature (T_b) in birds, approximately 39 to 42°C, evaporative heat loss is the only means of heat loss available to them.[1]

Birds lack sweat glands, and although evaporative heat loss through the skin has been shown to be significant in birds,[2] evaporation from the respiratory surfaces becomes the chief mode of thermoregulation for birds at high ambient temperatures. Respiratory evaporative heat loss (REHL) is proportional to the ventilation of the surface area available for evaporation and hence can be enhanced by increases in expired minute volume (V_E), whether these increases are effected by augmentation of tidal volume (V_T) or respiratory frequency (f). Menuam and Richards[3] have demonstrated a close proportionality between REHL and V_E in the chicken.

Almost all birds increase their REHL when needed by some form of "panting"; i.e., rapid, shallow breathing. Panting will be discussed in detail below. In some birds, panting is supplemented by "gular fluttering", i.e., rapid vibration of the floor of the buccal cavity. Lasiewski and Snyder[4] have described this response in detail. Blood flow to the buccal region is particularly enhanced during hyperthermia and movement of the moist gular area by action of the hyoid and tracheal muscles has been shown to contribute up to 20% of the total evaporative heat loss in the hyperthermic Quail (*Coturnix coturnix*)[5] and 35% in the Chicken (*Gallus gallus*).[6] Gular flutter frequencies are synchronous with panting frequency in some birds — for example, the Pigeon (*Columba livia*) — but in other species it is not.[2]

Gular fluttering is particularly advantageous in augmenting REHL since the energy expenditure is small and, unlike panting, gas exchange is not compromised.

One other interesting response observed in Doves which may contribute to increasing evaporative heat loss during hyperthermia is a rhythmic inflation of the esophagus.[7] Presumably, heat can be transferred from the warm blood of the subcutaneous vascular plexus in the cervical region to the esophageal membranes which are cooled by pulsating movements of the esophagus. This response seems to enhance thermoregulatory ability at high T_a in the Dove; whether it occurs in other birds needs to be studied.

B. Patterns of Panting
1. Normal Values for Maximal f during Panting

There is a wide range of respiratory patterns during hyperthermia among the various bird species and, hence, "panting" remains an ill-defined response. We choose to use "panting" in its broadest sense — merely, large increases in f which are accompanied, for the most part, by decreases in V_T. Generally, large birds such as the Ostrich (*Struthio camelus*),[8,9] Emu (*Dromaius novaehollandiae*),[10] or Swan (*Cygnus olar*).[11,12] pant at rather low maximal f (about 50 to 80 min^{-1}); these may be from 4 times[8] to 29 times[11] resting levels. The Pigeon, on the other hand, shows maximal panting f exceeding 600 min^{-1},[13-19] about 20 times that of rest. Calder and King[20] have calculated a general equation for the relationship between panting frequency and body mass for birds. Equations for doves and pigeons are similar to those obtained from data in panting mammals. Panting frequencies of other birds, however, are considerably lower than mammals of comparables sizes; this may be expected since resting f in birds are generally lower than in mammals.

2. "Resonant Panting" in Birds

It has been suggested[19,20] that some birds (for example, the Pigeon) pant at f equal to the resonant frequency of their respiratory system. That is, during hyperthermia panting f remains within relatively narrow limits, which is the optimal range in terms of minimal energy expenditure by expiratory muscles and maximum REHL. At resonant frequency, inertial and elastic resistive forces to flow are of equal magnitude but opposite phase so they cancel each other. Therefore, the only work needed to be performed is that of overcoming frictional resistance. Implicit in the "resonant panting" hypothesis is that panting is an all-or-none response, switching on immediately to a maximum f which is near the resonant frequency of the respiratory system. This is certainly not the case in the Chicken, where panting f varies, depending on the rise in T_b during hyperthermia.[21-27] Furthermore, Lacy[28] reports that experimentally induced increases in the elastance and inertance of the chest wall of panting Chickens, which should, respectively, increase and decrease the resonant frequency of chest-lung system, had no consistent effects on panting f.

On the other hand, Crawford and Kampe[19] claim supporting evidence for the concept of "resonant panting" in the Pigeon: the resonant frequency of the respiratory system of the Pigeon[29] was found to be near the f observed in some studies during panting in that species. However, several studies in the Pigeon[13-15,17,18] have shown that with a gradually ensuing hyperthermia, f rises gradually from resting levels to maximal panting. Figure 1 shows an example of how f in the Pigeon is related to T_a and duration of exposure. Therefore, it is certain that Pigeons do not always pant at resonant frequency. Of course, this does not exclude the possibility that maximum f during panting may be near resonant frequency. But, as Weathers[14] points out in examining the data of Crawford and Kampe,[19] although measured resonant frequency is near the maximal panting rates seen in Pigeons, no significant increase in energetic efficiency would be expected over a range in f of 240 to 840 br · min^{-1}. In mammalian studies, considerable breath-to-breath variation in f is usually seen during rest. Mead[30] suggests from studies in the guinea pig that "the cost of changes in respiratory

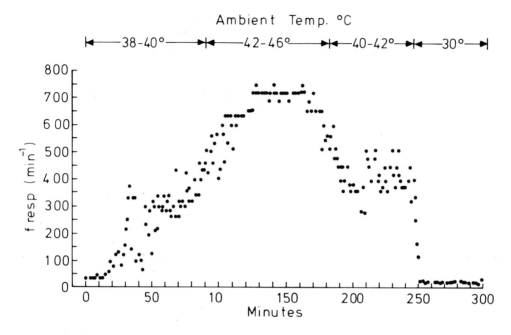

FIGURE 1.   Illustration of the dependency of respiratory frequency (f) of a Pigeon on ambient temperature (indicated at top) and duration of exposure to heating or cooling. Note that many intermediate respiratory frequencies are possible. (From Weathers, W. E., *J. Comp. Physiol.*, 79, 70, 1972. With permission.)

frequency over a wide range is remarkably little in terms of either respiratory work or muscle force." It remains to be seen whether f during maximal panting is regulated within strict limits in a given bird and, if so, whether this is advantageous to survival. Thus, "resonant panting" in birds it is yet to be confirmed as a physiological response and, in fact, does not seem to be necessarily useful in terms of minimizing the energy cost of REHL.

3. Dependency of f and VT on the Degree of Hyperthermia

Although there is evidence that some birds always pant at a discreet f, in most birds f increases gradually with a 1°C rise in T_b during exposure to high T_a and remains at a relatively stable plateau during a further 2 to 3°C rise in T_b. These plateaus are referred to as "phase 1 panting" and are accompanied by pronounced decreases in VT. Figure 2 shows examples of the typical responses of Chickens exposed to high T_a, and Figure 3 (X and open symbols) shows how increases in f are associated with decreases in VT. This latter relationship is such that, during phase 1 panting, VE is proportional to f. If REHL is not increased greatly enough during phase 1 panting, T_b will continue to rise. At some threshold T_b, VT begins to increase and f fall; for example, in Figure 2 after 1 hr at 40°C. It seems that the increase in VT actually preceeds the decline in f, and the resulting VE actually is enhanced.[27] This change in breathing pattern is usually referred to as "2nd phase" panting and may reflect a failure in the normal control mechanisms integrating physiological needs. Specifically, during 2nd phase panting, central mechanisms no longer guard against other consequences of great increase in VE, namely, pronounced imbalances in the acid-base status in the blood and, ultimately, fluid compartments in the body. Note that in Figure 3, points during 2nd phase panting (closed squares) do not seem to follow the relationship seen during phase 1 panting, suggesting that different central control mechanisms may be operating.

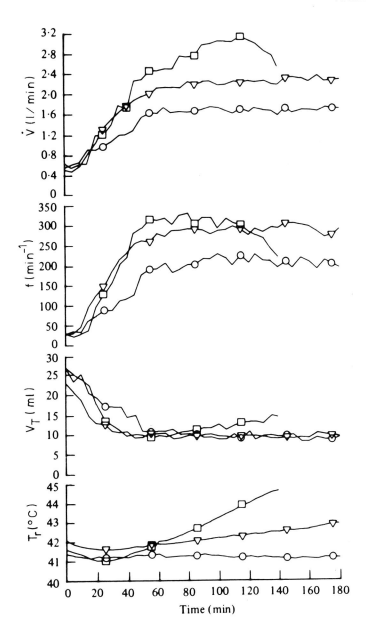

FIGURE 2.   Responses of minute volume (V̇), respiratory frequency (f), tidal volume (Vᴛ), and rectal temperature (Tᵣ) of Hens exposed to ambient temperatures of 30°C (○), 35°C (▽), and 40°C (□). Each point is a mean of five (30°C, 40°C) or eight (35°C) determinations. (From Kassim, H. and Sykes, A. H., *J. Exp. Biol.*, 97, 301, 1982. With permission.)

C. Acid-Base Balance during Hyperthermia
1. Hypocapnia and Its Consequences

Since the respiratory system also serves gas exchange, the need to augment V̇ᴇ and REHL in a hot environment may compromise the homeostasis of blood gases required for continued optimum physiological function. Changes in CO_2 partial pressure (PCO_2) in the blood will markedly affect acid-base balance because of its buffering properties: CO_2 is hydrated in the blood and then dissociates into H^+ and HCO_3^-. In fact, this CO_2-bicarbonate buffer

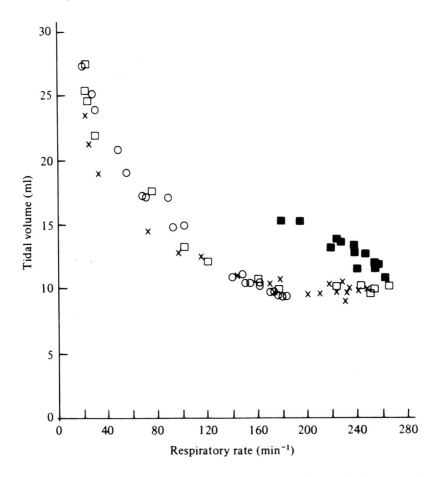

FIGURE 3.   Data from Figure 2 plotted to show the relationship between tidal volume and frequency of respiration in Hens exposed to ambient temperatures of 30°C (○), 35°C (X), and 40°C (□, Phase 1 panting; ■, second phase panting — i.e., after tidal volume increases from its minimum value). (From Kassim, H. and Sykes, A. H., *J. Exp. Biol.,* 97, 301, 1982. With permission.)

system is one of the most important ways in which the body regulates the pH of its fluids. Too much CO_2 results in acidoses (low pH) while, conversely, hypocapnia (low blood PCO_2) results in alkalosis. Arterial PCO_2 (Pa_{CO_2}) and pH (pHa) are usually used as indicators of the acid-base status of an animal and are inversely related in a way defined by the blood-buffer curve of the animal. After a prolonged panting episode, pHa may begin to decrease (return towards normal) even if hypocapnia remains. This is because the kidneys may effect a metabolic acidosis in order to compensate for the original alkalosis due to increased V_E.

The physiological repercussions of prolonged hypocapnia in birds need to be more fully studied. It is interesting to note that, unlike in mammals where hypocapnia severely restricts flow of blood in the brain, no cerebral vasoconstriction occurs in hypocapnic birds,[31,32] and cerebral blood flow may actually be enhanced by hyperthermia.[33] At least in this way, birds seem immune to one potential problem associated with increased V_E.

Birds, however, are prone to other consequences of hypocapnia. Since eggs and fowl meat are important worldwide sources of nourishment, there are important economical ramifications in understanding how birds control their acid-base balance. For example, alkalosis during high ambient temperature has been pointed to as a possible cause for the laying of low-quality eggs during hot summer months in some regions: lowering of H^+ and

HCO_3^- because of low CO_2 in the blood may severely inhibit eggshell deposition or otherwide restrict efficiency.[34,35]

Hypocapnia may also inhibit full expression of increase in V_E needed to combat hyperthermia, and therefore restrict growth and survival in hot climates. Birds, like mammals, have powerful receptor systems which sense CO_2 and act to inhibit respiration if CO_2 in the blood decreases. Birds possess central chemosensitivity to CO_2 as do mammals,[36] and have carotid bodies which are somewhat CO_2 sensitive.[37] In addition, birds have receptors in the lung, intrapulmonary chemoreceptors (IPC) which are remarkably sensitive to CO_2[38] and seem to inhibit tidal volume as CO_2 decreases from normal.[38-42] However, the reflex inhibition of V_E from chemoreceptors due to the need to prevent hypocapnia would seem to be in conflict with the thermoregulatory demand to augment V_E. Let use see how birds have been shown to deal with these conflicts of physiological interests.

2. Increases in $\dot{V}_E$, REHL and Gas Exchange

As discussed above, the increase in V_E during panting is mainly afforded by large increases in f with decreases in V_T. This diminishing of V_T ensures that the upper airways, especially, are ventilated at a great rate. A larger percentage of the volume of each breath will be confined to the respiratory dead space and, therefore, not reach the gas-exchange region of the lung. Menuam and Richards[3] have shown that most of the REHL in the chicken takes place in the upper airways. (This, incidentally, contrasts with the earlier assertions[43,44] that the air sacs are significant sites of heat loss. Those assertions may be true in the Ostrich, though, since, unlike the Chicken,[3] air sac temperatures are lower than core temperature during panting, and heat transfer to exhaled air would be facilitated.[8]) Thus, it would seem that panting is a respiratory-control mechanism that allows for simultaneous adjustments for thermoregulatory and gas-exchange demands.

3. Early Studies

Studies during the 1960s and early 1970s in birds during severe hyperthermia induced by a step increase in T_a to about 45°C reported pronounced hypocapnia during thermal panting.[23,25,45-49] These results are included in Table 1 but, unfortunately, reports of respiratory values are mostly lacking, and it is difficult to ascertain whether first or second phase panting was present. Thus, the severity of the hypocapnia in those studies may reflect very high levels of hyperthermia, not expected in birds exposed to daily fluctuations in T_a. The Ostrich seems an exception in regard to developing alkalosis: Schmidt-Nielsen et al.[8] report that they "observed no decrease in arterial P_{CO_2} during heat stress, even when Ostriches panted heavily for periods up to 8 hrs." They did not report any values for P_{CO_2}, but pHa measurements by Jones[9] in intensely panting Ostriches showed that only a mild alkalosis occurred, although he did not measure Pa_{CO_2}. Since Schmidt-Nielsen et al.[8] did find that intraclavicular air sac gas P_{CO_2}, which usually approximates the P_{CO_2} at the end of the gas-exchange region,[50] decreased from 42 to 13 torr from resting to panting in the Ostrich, it would seem that a large part of the enchanced V_E during panting is shunted away from gas-exchange regions to non-gas-exchanging sites such as the air sacs. In the case of the panting Ostrich, this would mean that tidal air flowed directly into the interclavicular air sac, without transiting the gas-exchange region and accumulating CO_2, as usually is the case.

4. "Shunting" of Gases away from the Gas-Exchange Region

The possibility of shunting of gases in the avian lung has been suggested by several authors[8,44] and has led to much discussion. Because of the unique arrangement of the bird's respiratory system,[51] it is easy to imagine how a shunting mechanism might work: changes in diameter of bronchial smooth muscle could conceivably redirect gas flows by changes in resistance to flow at certain critical points. For instance, Molony et al.[52] did find that low

Table 1

CHANGES IN RESPIRATORY FREQUENCY (f), PCO₂, AND pH IN THE ARTERIAL BLOOD ACCOMPANYING PANTING DURING EXPOSURES TO INCREASED AMBIENT TEMPERATURE IN BIRDS

Species	N	T_a (°C)	T_b (°C)	$f/f_c{}^a$	Pa_{CO_2} (torr)	$Pa_{CO_2} - Pa_{CO_2}C$ (torr)^a	pHa	pHa − pHa C^a	Comments	Ref.
Gallus domesticus										
White Leghorn ♂	3	45	42.5—44.5	9—10	22—18	−7—−11	7.56—7.61	0.05—0.10		23
White Leghorn ♂	6	40	43—45	—	15	−11	7.61—7.66	0.15—0.20		45
White Rock ♂	3	44	44.3	—	26	−3	7.53	0		48
Black Bantam ♀	2	50	—	—	14	−16	7.64	0.16		48
White Leghorn ♀	4	40	—	—	24	−3	7.54	0		49
North Holland Blue ♂	2	40	—	—	20	−9	7.53	0.05		49
White Leghorn ♂	19	45	42—43	7—8	19—18	−7—−8	7.55—7.60	0.6—0.11		25
Bedouin (Sinai) ♀	12 + 6	40 + 45	42.5 + 43.6	7	29 + 23	+1 + −6^b	7.57 + 7.58	0.04 + 0.05^b	Desert species	24
Bedouin (Beersheba) ♀	12 + 10	40 + 45	42.8 + 43.3	10	26 + 25	−2 + −3^b	7.53 + 7.54	−0.1 + 0^b	Desert species	24
Leghorn-Bedouin cross ♀	16 + 4	42 + 45	42.1 + 42.4	13 + 16	22 + 21	−2 + −3^b	7.56	0.01	Desert species cross; extensive acclimatization	56
Bedouin, White Leghorn and Crosses ♀	26	35—45	42—44	11—17	27—20^c	−2—−8	7.55—7.59	0.01—0.05		57
Breed not reported ♀	5	35—41	41.8—44.0	4—5	32—20	−4—−16	7.51—7.65	0.04—0.12		26
Breed not reported ♀	14	33	42.8	19	25	−4	7.54	0.06		58
White Leghorn-Rhode Island Red Cross ♀	6 + 7	Hot air blown at bird	42.5—43.3	4—6	24—22	−7—−9	7.48 + 7.46	0 + 0.02		33
Columba livia										
Pigeon	14	51	43.1	22	12	−16	7.69	0.17		46
	6	Gradual increase	43 + 44	10 + 18^d	26^e	0	7.50	0	Complete darkness	17
	6	Gradual increase	42.3—44.3	17—22	25—22^c	−3—−7	7.57—7.59	0.02—0.04		18
Anser platyrhynchos										
Pekin Duck	3	45	42	—	13	−17	7.7	0.20		48
	9	30 + 35	41.6 + 41.7	20 + 26	28 + 27^c	−2 + −3	7.52 — 7.53	0.02 + 0.03	Extensive training	59

Species									Notes	Ref
Struthio camelus										
Ostrich	20	39—56	39.9—40.2	7	Observed no decrease in Pa_{CO_2}[b,f]; no values given	—	—	—	Warm-weather species	8
Anser anser										
Goose	7	35 + 45	40.0 + 41.0	10	—	—	7.47	0.01	Warm-weather species	9
Cathartes aura										
Turkey Vulture	1	44	40.6	—	9	-16	7.76	0.23		48
	1	46	40.1	—	19	-9	7.56	0.05		48
Larus argentatus										
Herring Gull	1	43	—	—	10	-17	7.86	0.03		48
Geococcyx californianus										
Roadrunner	1	49	43.9	—	16	-9	7.71	0.13		48
Pelicanus erythrorhynchos										
White Pelican	3	46	41.1	10	19	-10	7.64	0.14		48
Spenorhynchus abdimii										
Abdim's Stork	5 + 9	40 + 45	40.4 + 41.1	10	27 + 26[g]	-2 + -3[a]	7.57	0.01	Warm-weather species	60
Alectorus chukar										
Rock Partridge	5 + 8	40 + 42	—	—	29 + 25[a]	+2 + -2[a]	7.54 + 7.56	0 + 0.02	Eyes covered, extensive training	61
Mute Swan	4	35	41.1	31	26	-1	7.56	0.06	Resting f = 3 min^{-1}	12
Pygorcelic adeliae, antartica, and papua										
Penguin	23	30—40	39.6—40.7	2—6	Inverse proportion to T_b + f			Proportional to T_b + f		63
Dromaius novaehollandiae										
Emu	2	46	39	10	30	-4	7.47	0.02	Warm-weather species	10

a   C means values of control at neutral ambient temperature.
b   Comparisons do not contain the same "N".
c   Calculated from reported linear regressions.
d   Fast component (see text) of respiratory pattern.
e   Report more severe hypocapnia at higher T_a.
f   Interclavicular air sac P_{CO_2} decreased from 42 to approximately 13 torr.
g   Report more severe hypocapnia in "restless birds." Pa_{CO_2} = 10 to 19 torr); values not included in table.

P_{CO_2} in artificially ventilated Ducks (*Anas platyrhynchos*) caused increased resistance to the flow of gas through the lung. The sites of this increase in resistance seemed to be the orifices of the medioventral secondary bronchi into the primary bronchus. However, Jones et al.[53] saw no changes in diameter of these orifices during the respiratory cycle, though air with virtually no CO_2 fills the airways on each inspiration. Also, Barnas et al.[54,55] did not find a significant response of smooth muscle in the Goose (*Anser anser*) lung to changes in P_{CO_2}, and Kampe and Crawford[29] found no change in airway resistance in Pigeons hyperventilated to the point of apnea. In summary, there is yet no conclusive evidence that birds can cause inhaled air to bypass their gas-exchange regions by alterations in smooth-muscle diameter in the lung in order to minimize hypocapnia during augmented $\dot{V}_E$.

5. Recent Studies

Most recent experiments in birds have verified that during hyperthermia the degree of hypocapnia is roughly proportional to the rise in T_b, as illustrated in Figure 4. During phase 1 panting, where T_b has not risen considerably, Pa_{CO_2} may only decrease a few torr. Therefore, panting can occur without severe hypocapnia, as seen in many studies in Table 1.[8-10,12,17,18,24,26,56-63] Note that several factors seem associated with minimizing hypocapnia during panting: (1) mild rises (to about 35°C) in T_a;[12,26,57,59,63] (2) genetic selection;[8,10,24,56,60] and (3) acclimatization.[59,61] Excitement also seems an important consideration since both Marder and Arad[60] and Krausz et al.[61] report that animals — not included in table averages — who were "restless" became very hypocapnic. It may be that excitement disrupts the ability of the respiratory-control system to maintain the balance between REHL and blood-gas homeostasis; alternately, excited birds may be increasing their heat production and therefore necessitate drastic REHL increases despite ensuing hypocapnia. The darkness during several of the experiments[17,61] may have contributed to minimalization of excitement. In addition, darkness has important effects on birds' thermoregulatory responses[64,65] and may be a factor in altering responsiveness to the heat stress.

6. Mechanisms That Prevent Severe Hypocapnia in Panting Birds

As suggested by Bech and Johansen,[12] no shunting mechanism is necessary to explain eucapnic panting in birds if the decrease in $\dot{V}_T$ during panting is such that mostly only tracheal dead space is being ventilated. In other words, the "effective minute ventilation", that part which actually reaches the gas-exchange area, may not be appreciably increased although $\dot{V}_E$ may increase greatly. For example, Figure 5 shows respiratory data from four breeds of Chicken over a range of T_a; note Pa_{CO_2} decreases as $\dot{V}_E$ is enhanced, especially as $\dot{V}_T$ increases from its minimum. Figure 6 shows that Pa_{CO_2} is inversely proportional to the percent of $\dot{V}_T$ compared to tracheal dead-space volume (Vtr). There are not yet sufficient data available to make similar analysis in other species, but the tendency to minimize increases in gas exchange during panting by preferentially ventilating dead space may help explain the cases in Table 1 where severe hypocapnia was prevented.

Although panting is manifested generally by increased f and decreased $\dot{V}_T$, breathing patterns may also show complex, periodic changes during a given hyperthermic episode, as reported in the Flamingo (*Phoenicopterus ruber*).[62] In those experiments, a "flush-out" pattern of ventilation was observed, where fast, shallow breathing is interrupted by intermittent, deep breaths. This type of ventilation was also observed in the Chicken and attributed to the buildup of CO_2 in the caudal air sacs and the consequent augmentation of $\dot{V}_T$ via intrapulmonary chemoreceptors.[67] This is supported by measurements of intraclavicular and abdominal air sac P_{CO_2} measurements in panting Chicken: the former decreases during panting (reflecting a lower Pa_{CO_2}), while the latter increases, indicating that very little of the fresh tidal air reaches the caudal air sacs.[67] Another pattern of panting, called "compound panting", was reported in the Pigeon.[16,17] In compound panting, deep, slow breaths (3 mℓ,

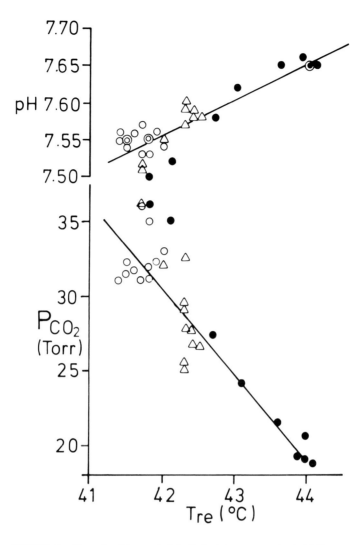

FIGURE 4. Example of how arterial pH (top) increases and arterial P_{CO_2} (bottom) decreases with a rise in rectal temperature (T_{re}) in Chickens. Ambient temperature was 35°C (○), 38°C (△), or 41°C (●). Each point is the mean of observations on five Hens; coincident points are circled. (From Hadi, E. El. and Sykes, A. H., *Br. Poult. Sci.*, 23, 49, 1982. With permission.)

20 min^{-1}) are superimposed on shallow, fast breaths (1 mℓ, 200 to 500 min^{-1}). The shallow breaths approximate the tracheal dead space of the Pigeon and therefore should not contribute to gas exchange, which is maintained by the deeper breaths. In those studies Pa_{CO_2} remained stable until very high increases in T_b. Whether other species of birds also exhibit "compound panting" is not known, although it has been reported in sheep.[68]

In summary, panting is an illustration of how the respiratory system adapts to conflicting needs of gas exchange and thermoregulation. It seems likely that many birds are able to adjust their respiratory pattern during mild hyperthermia to increase $\dot{V}E$ without greatly disturbing acid-base balance. Severe hyperthermia, however, causes a pronounced hypocapnia as $\dot{V}T$ begins to increase from minimum levels, indicating second phase panting. The only exception so far seems to be the Ostrich which, as mentioned above, is reported to incur no severe alkalosis, even during intense panting where $\dot{V}T$ may increase above control.[8,9]

It should be mentioned here, however, that the idea that minimizing $\dot{V}T$ towards dead-

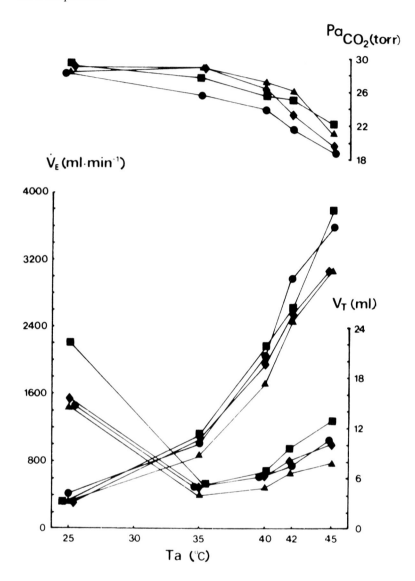

FIGURE 5. Effect of ambient temperature (T_a) on tidal volume (V_T) and minute volume (V_E) on four breeds of Chickens; coincident changes in arterial P_{CO_2} (Pa_{CO_2}) indicated in upper section. Breeds are Sinai (▲), Leghorn (●), Sinai-Leghorn cross (■), and Leghorn-Sinai cross (◆). Note that above 35°C, V_T increases from its minimum and Pa_{CO_2} decreases in all breeds, indicating 2nd phase panting (From Arad, Z. and Marder, J., *Comp. Biochem. Physiol.*, 74A, 125, 1983. With permission.)

space volume prevents all but essential gas exchange and minimizes hypocapnia may be too simplistic, especially considering the high f seen in some panting birds. If such a mechanism were to operate, gas exchange would theoretically be zero if V_T equals V_{tr}. As can be seen in Figure 6, even when V_T is less than 100% V_{tr}, sufficient CO_2 is lost to prevent large increases in Pa_{CO_2}. It has been demonstrated in mammals that artificial high-frequency ventilation (HFV) of the lungs by respiratory pumps at frequencies of 1 to 60 Hz can maintain gas exchange even when the pump volumes are much less than tracheal dead-space volume.[69] Recently, Banzett and Lehr[70] used HFV on chickens. Their results indicate that significant CO_2 elimination occurs even if pump volumes are 30% of dead-space volume when pump frequencies are greater than 2 Hz. At higher frequencies, up to 15 Hz, CO_2 elimination

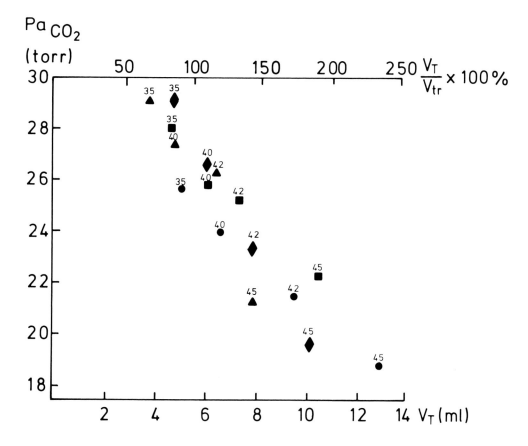

FIGURE 6.   Data from Figure 5 plotted to illustrate how arterial P_{CO_2} (Pa_{CO_2}) at various ambient temperatures (indicated above symbols) is related to tidal volume (V_T) or its fraction of predicted tracheal volume (V_T/V_{tr}). Symbols same as Figure 5; V_{tr} predicted from Reference 56. (From Arad, Z. and Marder, J., *Comp. Biochem. Physiol.*, 74A, 125, 1983. With permission.)

proportionally increases. Thus, other factors may also be involved with minimizing hypocapnia in panting birds even when V_T is near tracheal dead-space volume.

One of these possible factors may be the effect of panting on the hypothesized "aerodynamic valving" (see Chapter 2) that directs flow through the avian lung. Not much is actually known about the characteristics of these proposed "valves". Are they affected by high flow rates, such as are present during panting? Do the high frequencies present during panting affect their function? Although Bretz and Schmidt-Nielsen[71] report that, generally, flow through the Duck lung during submaximal panting is the same as at rest, small inefficiencies of aerodynamic valving could conceivably change flows (e.g., shunt air from trachea directly to cranial air sac) and affect gas exchange. In fact, preliminary results[72] show that the efficiency of the aerodynamic valving of the Goose lung is affected by factors which may be important during panting such as flow velocity and flow periods. More thorough investigations of aerodynamic valves and their characteristics in controlling air flow in the avian lung need to be made. Perhaps the ability of some birds to resist hypocapnia during severe hyperthermia may be partly attributable to changing flow patterns during panting.

D. Control of Panting

1. Central and Peripheral Neural Influences

Although an intact hypothalamus is essential for proper thermoregulatory responses in birds to a cold or warm environment,[73,74] its role in the control of panting has not been clearly evaluated. Inputs to the respiratory center from other regions, especially from the midbrain and spinal cord, seem more powerful in evoking panting, and panting can occur without an intact hypothalamus in birds,[75,76] if the rise in T_b is sufficient.

A "panting center" where electrical stimulation elicits breathing similar to thermally induced panting is well documented in Pigeons[13,76] and Chickens.[76] This center is located in the dorsal midbrain and may be analogous to the pneumotaxic center in mammals[75-77] (see Chapter 10). Although medullary stimulation after transection of this panting center can cause increase in f, breathing then is much slower and deeper than normal panting.

The importance of hypothalamic thermosensitivity is minimal in birds. Rather, thermoreceptors in the spinal cord are predominant in determining thermoregulatory responses.[78-81] Heating the spinal cord alone can cause immediate panting in Pigeons while cooling the cord will immediately inhibit panting induced by ambient heating. All respiratory and cardiovascular changes induced by such spinal-cord temperature manipulations are very similar to responses seen when whole-body temperature is altered.[18] Peripheral thermosensitivity is also important in the bird, especially as a modulator of responses caused by internal body-temperature changes.[82,83]

Afferent neural information in the vagus nerves is important in determining breathing patterns during hyperthermia. In all avian species studied, sectioning of one vagus during hyperthermic panting reduced f slightly and, in all species except the Pigeon, bilateral vagotomy abolished rapid breathing during hyperthermia.[84,85] Electrical stimulation of the cut central ends of the vagi in the Chicken reinstated panting.[85] Although the Pigeon, unlike all other species tested, was able to pant after bilateral vagotomy, f at a given increase in T_b was lower than compared to Pigeons with intact vagi.

In summary, in terms of thermoregulation, the hypothalamus should be considered an integrator of inputs from the spinal cord, brain, and periphery and not the sole controller of thermoregulatory response. The question remains as to how the panting response is controlled to balance gas exchange and thermoregulatory needs.

2. Influence of CO_2 on Panting

It has been suggested that hypocapnia may be a necessary part of the normal panting response. Supporting evidence for the involvement of hypocapnia in the control of thermal panting has been shown in the awake Chicken: prevention of alkalosis during severe hyperthermia by CO_2 supplementation of the inhaled air decreased panting frequencies while tidal volume was enhanced.[25] Such an inhibition of f during panting by CO_2, in contrast to its normally f-increasing effect, has also been reported in the Chicken by Richards and Avery,[75] Barnas et al.,[86,87] and Brackenbury,[88] and in the Pigeon by Saalfeld,[13] and is referred to as a "paradoxical effect" of CO_2 on f — i.e., increasing at normal T_b, decreasing at high T_b. It is also interesting to note that Saalfeld[13] and Mather et al.[25] report an overall increase in $\dot{V}E$ during CO_2 supplement while panting occurred, since VT was enhanced. This would seem to suggest that when the need to minimize hypocapnia is abolished (i.e., CO_2 is available in the air), $\dot{V}E$ can increase more readily in response to thermoregulatory needs. This would have important consequences economically. Perhaps CO_2 supplementation would enhance the $\dot{V}E$ of poultry in hot summer months; REHL would be increased and the birds would be better able to withstand the heat stress.

More information about how the respiratory system of birds acts to serve both thermoregulatory and gas-exchange needs is provided by experiments employing the technique of artificial unidirectional ventilation, which is afforded by the unique structure of the avian

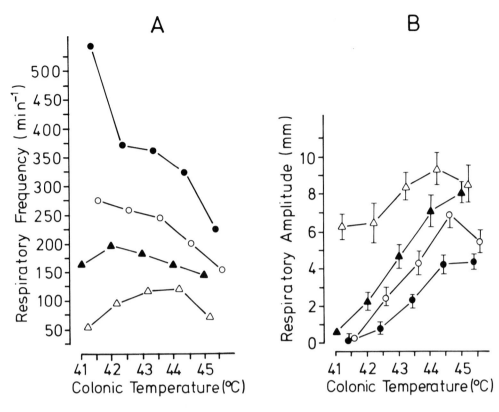

FIGURE 7. Respiratory frequencies (A) and amplitude (B) of six anesthetized, unidirectionally ventilated Cockerels during rising colonic temperature. In such preparations arterial Pco_2 is almost exactly equal to Pco_2 of the ventilatory gas which was 7 torr (●), 14.0 torr (○), 21 torr (▲), or 35 torr (△). Note that below 35 torr Pco_2, respiratory frequency decreases with colonic temperature, and respiratory amplitude increases with colonic temperature at all Pco_2. (From Barnas, G. M., Estavillo, J. A., Mather, F. B., and Burger, R. E., *Respir. Physiol.*, 43, 315, 1981. With permission.)

respiratory system. Warm, humid air, containing exact levels of CO_2, is flowed through the trachea, over the lungs, and out of a cannulated air sac. Or conversely, flow is from air sac, through the lungs, and out the mouth. Gas exchange during unidirectional flow in either direction is very efficient and, by adjusting to the level of CO_2 in the gas, Pa_{CO_2} can be precisely adjusted. At normal Pa_{CO_2} (about 35 torr), f increases only to about 100 min^{-1} during hyperthermia in the unidirectionally ventilated Chicken, well below the normal of 240 min^{-1} (Figure 7A). When Pa_{CO_2} is kept constant at hypocapnic levels (7 to 21 torr) and T_b is made to rise, f actually decreases as T_b rises ("paradoxical effect"). At any constant level of Pa_{CO_2}, V_T increases as T_b increases (Figure 7B). Similar results have also been seen in the Pigeon.[89] Thus, the thermoregulatory drive is such that V_T is increased by hyperthermia and f generally decreases. This effect is independent of whether the input from chemoreceptors is from the lungs alone (IPC) or from systemic chemoreceptors.[87] Brackenbury and Gleeson[90] also found evidence in awake, unrestrained Chickens that decreases in Pa_{CO_2} are important in the normal panting response. Closed triangles in Figure 8 show that, in response to an increase in T_a to 35°C, V_T decreases as f greatly increases (note inverse scale for f). These changes were accompanied by a 2- to 3-torr fall in interclavicular air sac Pco_2. If Pco_2 was kept constant at 37 torr by adding CO_2 to the inhaled gas, f rose only to 60 min^{-1} and V_T increased. They concluded that only a 2- to 3-torr fall in Pa_{CO_2} may be sufficient to exert a powerful influence on the respiratory pattern. Such a mild hypocapnia has been

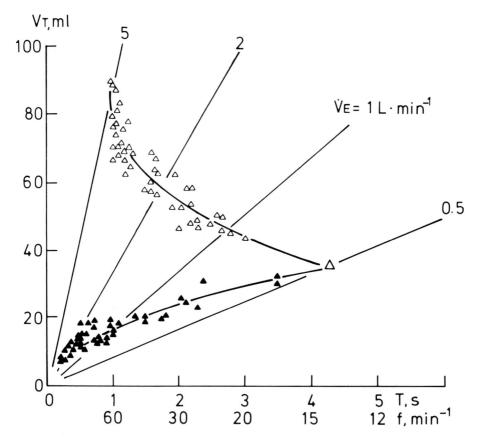

FIGURE 8. Progressive changes in respiratory pattern induced by increasing ambient temperature from 18 to 35°C in Chickens under normal conditions (▲) and when hypocapnia is prevented (△). Large open triangle in right of figure denotes resting conditions. Normally during hyperthermia, minute volume ($\dot{V}E$) increases (leftward shift through isominute volume lines) as respiratory frequency (f) increases and tidal volume (V_T) decreases; decreases in P_{CO_2} in the lung are concurrent with these changes. If CO_2 is added, maximum f is much lower than normal. (From Brackenbury, J. H. and Gleeson, M., *Respir. Physiol.,* 54, 109, 1983. With permission.)

measured in an overwhelming percentage of the experiments studying mild panting (Table 1) and may be important, in most cases, in determining respiratory responses to hyperthermia. Thus, feedback from central and peripheral (carotid bodies and IPC) CO_2 receptors probably contributes to the control of panting to balance thermoregulatory and gas-exchange needs.

III. RESPIRATION DURING HYPOTHERMIA

A. Respiration Accompanying Specific Hypothermic States

All birds investigated so far show a pronounced circadian rhythm of body temperature.[65] The amplitude of fluctuation depends on body size and T_a. Pigeons weighing about 0.4 kg have an amplitude of 3 to 4°C between day and night at T_a of 5°C.[64] Our own unpublished observations in this species indicated a reduction in f of 10 to 15% in the nightly sleeping state, where T_b was lowered. The reduction of f was closely correlated with the depression of shivering thermogenesis and decreases in metabolic rate. No reports exist at the present time on changes in V_T, $\dot{V}E$, blood gases, or pH during slow-wave and rapid-eye-movement sleep states in avian species.

Torpor is a deep hypothermia in endothermic animals in which body temperature falls by

10 to 15°C below normal level. This phenomenon takes place seasonally in most Nightjars (Caprimulgidae) and daily during night phase in small birds (less than 15 g) at low T_a. Metabolism, heart frequency, and f decrease with decreasing T_b,[91] but V_T and V_E have not been measured, perhaps owing to difficulties in obtaining these measurements in such small animals.

B. Respiration during Shivering Thermogenesis

1. Control of Shivering

During a lowering of T_a, birds must increase their internal heat production in order to protect against hypothermia.[1,77,81,91,92] The effector mechanism of this heat production is shivering, a tremor of the skeletal muscles, which produces heat but no locomotion.[93] Shivering, as in voluntary muscle work, is always accompanied by increasing oxygen uptake. Rautenberg[94] found a close relationship between tremor intensity and oxygen consumption in Pigeons. No clear evidence of any kind of nonshivering thermogenesis have been reported in birds, though this phenomenon is well demonstrated in many mammalian species.[95]

The cold tremor of birds can be evoked by lowering of T_a and by selective cooling of the CNS, especially the spinal cord.[78,79,96] This kind of thermal stimulation effects the same responses in shivering and oxygen consumption as ambient cooling.[96] Important thermo-detectors are obviously concentrated in the spinal cord of birds.[81,97-99] Cooling the spinal cord of Pigeons at neutral T_a evokes vigorous shivering within a few seconds, whereas lowering T_a causes a slow increase in shivering intensity as skin temperature slowly decreases.[78,79,83]

2. Increases in Respiration Accompanying Shivering

In Pigeons[100,101] and Fish Crows (*Corvus assifragus*),[102] increases in V_E are closely correlated with increases in heat production caused by shivering. An example of ventilatory responses in Pigeons is shown in Figure 9 A through C: V_T, f, and V_E increase with heat production (M) during cold stimulations. Oxygen extraction from the inhaled gas [E_{O_2} = (V_{O_2} × 100)/(V_I × 0.2095)] remained relatively constant when M increased in Pigeons and Crows (*Corvus corone*) (Figure 10). In some other avian species — Pekin Duck (*Anas platyrhynchos*),[103] Kittiwake (*Rissa tridactyla*),[104] and Coot (*Fulica atra*)[105] — divergence was found between M and V_E, and E_{O_2}, M_{O_2} increased at low T_a. Johansen and Bech[106] interpreted these results as a minimalization of REHL under cold conditions. That is, at low T_a, it would be advantageous for the bird to retain heat by ventilating less for a given amount of O_2 consumed. We are unsure at this time whether these differences in respiratory responses depend on species or experimental methods. Bech and Rautenberg[109] recently repeated experiments in the Pigeon using the same method as those studies in which E_{O_2} increased at low T_a and found, again, that E_{O_2}, was constant in the Pigeons. Further investigations of various species may clarify this question of whether respiration is controlled in the cold to serve thermoregulation in addition to matching O_2 demands.

3. Control of Respiration during Shivering

The fact that spinal-cord cooling evokes shivering in a few seconds at neutral T_a allows us a method to investigate the dynamic courses of tremor and ventilation.[100] V_T and f increase immediately with the start of muscle tremor. The same fast response of ventilation is reported for physical muscle work in mammalian species (cf. DiMarco et al.[107]). DiMarco et al.[107] have shown that the immediate changes of ventilatory pattern can be generated both by afferent nervous signals coming from muscle proprioreceptors and efferents coming from locomotor centers in the brainstem. The same appears to be in case for shivering.[100] The importance of chemical information in ventilatory control can be excluded at the starting

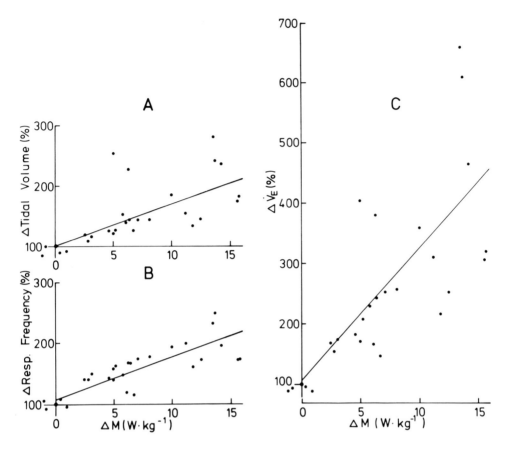

FIGURE 9.   Relationships of percentage changes in (A) tidal volume, (B) respiratory frequency, and (C) expired volume (V̇E) to increases in heat production (M) in five Pigeons exposed to spinal-cord and/or ambient coolings. Linear regressions indicated by solid lines. (From Barnas, G. and Rautenberg, W., *Pflügers Arch.*, 401, 228, 1984. With permission.)

phase of muscle activity since a time delay would necessarily occur. This would not be true during the course of persistent exercise or shivering.

4. Blood Gases during Shivering

Studies of blood gases and pH during shivering were made in Pigeons[100,101] and Pekin Ducks.[103] The two species showed no dramatic alteration of arterial and mixed venous pH and PCO_2 during shivering, though a trend for PCO_2 to increase was observed. The increase, however, was not well correlated to the increase of heat production. Mixed venous PO_2 and O_2 content (CO_2) decreased significantly during shivering in Pigeons, and the arterial-venous differences in PO_2 and CO_2 were closely related to increases in heat production caused by shivering.[100,108] However, in Pekin Ducks, mixed venous PO_2 and CO_2 increased during shivering in cold conditions,[103] and the arterial-venous differences did not change. These divergent results suggest that further studies in various avian species are required.

IV. SUMMARY

1.   Birds have not developed any anatomical structures specialized only to serve thermoregulation. As a result, the respiratory system may be called upon to function simultaneously in the regulations of body temperature and gas exchange. At times, these functions may be at odds.

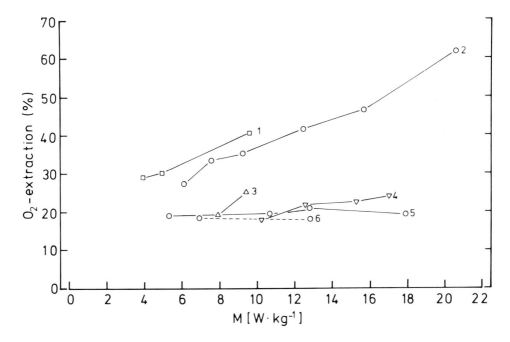

FIGURE 10.   Oxygen extraction in relation to heat production (M) during rest (right-most point of each curve) and shivering. Data from (1) Pekin Duck,[103] (2) Coot,[105] (3) Kittiwake,[104] (4) Crow,[102] (5) Pigeon,[100] and (6) Pigeon.[101]

2.   Panting (*viz;* fast shallow breathing) is the most important means of thermoregulation for birds during high temperatures. This is supplemented by "gular fluttering" in some species.

3.   There is no good evidence that birds pant at the resonant frequency of their respiratory system.

4.   Respiratory evaporative heat loss (REHL) is proportional to $\dot{V}E$. As T_b increases, $\dot{V}E$ is augmented by large increases, in f although $\dot{V}T$ is diminished (phase 1 panting). With further increases in T_b, $\dot{V}T$ begins to increase towards normal and f decreases (2nd phase panting).

5.   Only mild hypocapnia (decreases in blood P_{CO_2}) accompanies phase 1 panting, while severe hypocapnia usually is observed during 2nd phase panting.

6.   The ability of most birds to develop only slight hypocapnia while panting during mild hyperthermia is afforded by the respiratory control system which adjusts $\dot{V}T$ to balance REHL and gas-exchange (although other factors, i.e., air flow patterns in the lung, may be important).

7.   It is suggested that CO_2-receptors are important with controlling breathing during panting.

8.   More research is needed to understand the factors influencing respiration in birds which limit growth, egg production, and survival during hyperthermia.

9.   In cold environments, birds must increase their heat production by shivering; no evidence for nonshivering thermogenesis in birds has been found.

10.   Shivering can be evoked by either central or peripheral cooling. In birds, spinal-cord cooling is especially effective and shivering can be induced within seconds. Increases in $\dot{V}E$ always accompany shivering, whether it ensues gradually or immediately.

11.   In some species, the increase in $\dot{V}E$ accompanying shivering is well correlated with the increase in heat production: therefore, O_2 extraction (E_{O_2}) is constant during a

wide range of cold stress. In other species, EO_2 increases at low T_a, presumably to minimize REHL.

12. Changes in blood PCO_2 and pH are small during shivering; there have been conflicting reports concerning blood PO_2.

13. More research is needed concerning respiration in cold environments in birds. Specifically, questions concerning the importance of species differences in EO_2 and blood gases in the cold must be resolved. Additionally, such studies offer the opportunity for better insight into the relationship between VE and O_2 consumption when movement is minimal.

REFERENCES

1. **Whittow, G. C.,** Regulation of body temperature, in *Avian Physiology,* Sturkie, P. D., Ed., Springer-Verlag, Berlin, 1976, chap. 7.
2. **Dawson, W. R.,** Evaporative losses of water by birds, *Comp. Biochem. Physiol.,* 71A, 495, 1982.
3. **Menuam, B. and Richards, S. A.,** Observation on the sites of respiratory evaporation in the fowl during thermal panting, *Respir. Physiol.,* 25, 39, 1975.
4. **Lasiewski, R. C. and Snyder, G. K.,** Responses to high temperature in nestling double-crested and pelagic cormorants, *Auk,* 86, 529, 1969.
5. **Weathers, W. W. and Schoenbaechler, D. C.,** Contribution of gular flutter to evaporative cooling in Japanese quail, *J. Appl. Physiol.,* 40, 521, 1976.
6. **Brackenbury, J. H., Avery, P., and Gleeson, M.,** Respiratory evaporation in panting flow: partition between the respiratory and buccopharyngeal pumps, *J. Comp. Physiol.,* 145, 63, 1981.
7. **Gaunt, S. L.,** Thermoregulation in doves (*Columbidae*): a novel esophageal heat exchanger, *Science,* 210, 445, 1980.
8. **Schmidt-Nielsen, K., Kanwisher, J., Lasiewski, R. C., Cohn, J. E., and Bretz, W. L.,** Temperature regulation and respiration in the ostrich, *Condor,* 71, 341, 1969.
9. **Jones, J. H.,** Pulmonary blood flow distribution in panting ostriches, *J. Appl. Physiol.: Respirat. Environ. Exercise Physiol.,* 53(6), 1511, 1982.
10. **Jones, J. H., Gubb, B., and Schmidt-Nielsen, K.,** Panting in the emu causes arterial hypoxemia, *Respir. Physiol.,* 54, 189, 1983.
11. **Bech, C. and Johansen, K.,** Ventilation and gas exchange in the mute swan, *(Cygnus olor), Respir. Physiol.,* 39, 285, 1980.
12. **Bech, D. and Johansen, K.,** Ventilatory and circulatory responses to hyperthermia in the mute swan, *(Cygnus olor), J. Exp. Biol.,* 88, 195, 1980.
13. **Saalfeld, E. V.,** Untersuchungen über das Hacheln bei Tauben, *Z. Vl. Physiol.,* 23, 727, 1936.
14. **Weathers, W. E.,** Thermal panting in domestic pigeons, *Columba livia,* and the barn owl, *Tyoto alba, J. Comp. Physiol.,* 79, 70, 1972.
15. **Smith, R. M.,** Circulation, respiratory volumes and temperature regulation of the pigeon in dry and humid heat, *Comp. Biochem. Physiol.,* 43A, 477, 1972.
16. **Ramirez, J. M. and Bernstein, M. H.,** Compound ventilation during thermal panting in pigeons: a possible mechanism for minimizing hypocapnic alkalosis, *Fed. Proc. Fed. Am. Soc. Exp. Biol.,* 35, 2562, 1976.
17. **Bernstein, M. H. and Samaniego, F. C.,** Ventilation and acid-base status during thermal panting in pigeons, *(Columba livia), Physiol. Zool.,* 54, 303, 1981.
18. **Barnas, G. M. and Rautenberg, W.,** Cardiovascular and blood gas changes during panting responses induced by ambient or spinal cord heating in the pigeon, *Respir. Physiol.,* 57, 89, 1984.
19. **Crawford, E. C. and Kampe, G.,** Resonant panting in pigeons, *Comp. Biochem. Physiol.,* 40, 549, 1971.
20. **Calder, W. A. and King, J. R.,** Thermal and caloric relations of birds, in *Avian Biology,* Vol. 4, Farner, D. S. and King, J. R., Eds., Academic Press, New York, 1974, 259.
21. **Randall, W. C. and Hiestand, W. A.,** Panting and temperature regulation in the chicken, *Am. J. Physiol.,* 127, 761, 1939.
22. **Frankel, H., Hollands, K. G., and Weiss, H. S.,** Respiratory and circulatory responses of hyperthermic chickens, *Arch. Int. Physiol. Biochem.,* 70(4), 555, 1962.
23. **Linsley, J. G. and Burger, R. E.,** Respiratory and cardiovascular responses in the hyperthermic domestic cock, *Poult. Sci.,* 43, 292, 1964.

24. **Marder, J., Arad, Z., and Gafni, M.,** The effect of high ambient temperature on acid-base balance of panting Bedouin fowl *(Gallus domesticus), Physiol. Zool.,* 47, 180, 1974.
25. **Mather, R. B., Barnas, G. M., and Burger, R. E.,** The influence of alkalosis on panting, *Comp. Biochem. Physiol.,* 67(A), 265, 1980.
26. **Hadi, E. El and Sykes, A. H.,** Thermal panting and respiratory alkalosis in the laying hen, *Br. Poult. Sci.,* 23, 49, 1982.
27. **Kassim, H. and Sykes, A. H.,** The respiratory responses of the fowl to hot climates, *J. Exp. Biol.,* 97, 301, 1982.
28. **Lacy, R. A., Jr.,** Mechanical Determinants of Panting Frequency in the Domestic Fowl, thesis, University of California, Davis, 1965.
29. **Kampe, G. and Crawford, E. C.,** Oscillatory mechanics of the respiratory system of pigeons, *Respir. Physiol.,* 18, 188, 1973.
30. **Mead, J.,** Control of respiratory frequency, *J. Appl. Physiol.,* 15(3), 325, 1960.
31. **Grubb, B., Mills, C. D., Colacino, J. M., and Schmidt-Nielsen, K.,** Effect of arterial carbon dioxide on cerebral blood flow in ducks, *Am. J. Physiol.,* 232(6), H596, 1977.
32. **Wolfenson, D., Frei, Y. F., and Berman, A.,** Blood flow distribution during artificially induced respiratory hypocapnic alkalosis in the fowl, *Respir. Physiol.,* 50, 87, 1982.
33. **Wolfenson, D., Frei, Y. F., Sanpir, N., and Berman, A.,** Heat stress effects on capillary blood flow and its redistribution in the laying hen, *Pflügers Arch.,* 390, 86, 1981.
34. **Mongin, P.,** Role of acid-base balance in the physiology of egg shell formation, *World's Poult. Sci. J.,* 24, 200, 1968.
35. **Mongin, P.,** Acid-base balance during eggs shell formation, in *Respiratory Function in Birds, Adult and Embryonic,* Piiper, J., Ed., Springer-Verlag, Berlin, 1978, 247.
36. **Sebert, P.,** Mise en evidence de l'action centrale du stimulus CO_2-(H^+) de la ventilation chez le Canard Pekin, *J. Physiol. (Paris),* 75, 901, 1979.
37. **Bouverot, P.,** Control of breathing in birds compared with mammals, *Physiol. Rev.,* 58, 604, 1978.
38. **Peterson, D. F. and Fedde, M. R.,** Receptors sensitive to carbon dioxide in lungs of chicken, *Science,* 162, 1499, 1968.
39. **Osborne, J. L., Mitchell, G. S., and Powell, F.,** Ventilatory responses to CO_2 in the chicken: intrapulmonary and systemic chemoreceptors, *Respir. Physiol.,* 30, 369, 1977.
40. **Osborne, J. L. and Mitchell, G. S.,** Intrapulmonary and systemic CO_2-chemoreceptor interaction in the control of avian respiration, *Respir. Physiol.,* 33, 349, 1978.
41. **Burger, R. E. and Estavillo, J. A.,** The alteration of CO_2 sensitivity in chickens by thoracic visceral denervation, *Respir. Physiol.,* 32, 251, 1978.
42. **Burger, R. E., Barker, M. R., Nye, P. C. G., and Powell, F. L.,** Effects of intrapulmonary chemoreceptors in perfused and non-perfused lungs, in *Respiratory Function in Birds, Adult and Embryonic,* Piiper, J., Ed., Springer-Verlag, Berlin, 1978, 156.
43. **Salt, G. W. and Zeuthern, E.,** The respiratory system, in *Biology and Comparative Physiology of Birds,* Marshall, A. J., Ed., Academic Press, New York, 1960, chap. 10.
44. **Salt, G. W.,** Respiratory evaporation in birds, *Biol. Rev.,* 39, 113, 1964.
45. **Frankel, H. M. and Frascell, D.,** Blood respiratory gases, lactate and pyruvate during thermal stress in the chicken, *Proc. Soc. Exp. Biol. Med.,* 127, 997, 1968.
46. **Calder, W. A. and Schmidt-Nielsen, K.,** Evaporative cooling and respiratory alkalosis in the pigeon, *Proc. Natl. Acad. Sci. U.S.A.,* 55, 750, 1966.
47. **Calder, W. A. and Schmidt-Nielsen, K.,** Temperature regulation and evaporation in the pigeon and the roadrunner, *Am. J. Physiol.,* 213, 883, 1967.
48. **Calder, W. A. and Schmidt-Nielsen, K.,** Panting and blood carbon dioxide in birds, *Am. J. Physiol.,* 215, 477, 1968.
49. **Kampen, M., van,** Lung ventilation, pH, Pco_2 of arterial blood in the domestic fowl, Proc. 15th World Poultry Congr., New Orleans, August 11 to 16, 1974, 527.
50. **Brackenbury, J. H.,** Airflow and respired gases within the lung-air-sac system of birds, *Comp. Biochem. Physiol.,* 68(A), 1, 1981.
51. **King, A. S. and Cowie, A. F.,** The functional anatomy of the bronchial muscle of the bird, *J. Anat.,* 105, 323, 1969.
52. **Molony, V., Graf, W., and Scheid, P.,** Effects of CO_2 on pulmonary air flow resistance in the duck, *Respir. Physiol.,* 26, 333, 1976.
53. **Jones, J. H., Effmann, E. L., and Schmidt-Nielsen, K.,** Control of air flow in bird lungs, radiographic studies, *Respir. Physiol.,* 45, 121, 1981.
54. **Barnas, G. M., Mather, F. B., and Fedde, M. R.,** Response of avian intrapulmonary smooth muscle to changes in carbon dioxide concentration, *Poult. Sci.,* 57(5), 1400, 1978.
55. **Barnas, G. M., Mather, F. B., and Fedde, M. R.,** Are avian intrapulmonary CO_2 receptors chemically modulated mechanoreceptor or chemoreceptors?, *Respir. Physiol.,* 35, 237, 1978.

56. **Arad, Z., Moskovits, E., and Marder, J.,** A preliminary study of egg production and heat tolerance in a new breed of fowl (Leghorn × Bedouin), *Poult. Sci.,* 54, 780, 1975.

57. **Arad, Z. and Marder, J.,** Acid-base regulation during thermal panting in the fowl (*Gallus domesticus*): comparison between breeds, *Comp. Biochem. Physiol.,* 74A, 125, 1983.

58. **Gleeson, M. and Brackenbury, J. H.,** Ventilation, gaseous exchange and air sac gases during moderate thermal panting in domestic fowl, *Q. J. Exp. Physiol.,* 68, 591, 1983.

59. **Bouverot, B., Hildwein, G., and Legoff, D.,** Evaporative water loss, respiratory pattern, gas exchange and acid-base balance during thermal panting in Pekin ducks exposed to moderate heat, *Respir. Physiol.,* 21, 255, 1974.

60. **Marder, J. and Arad, Z.,** The acid base balance of Abdim's stork (*Sphenorhynchus abdimis*) during thermal panting, *Comp. Biochem. Physiol.,* 51A, 887, 1975.

61. **Krausz, S., Bernstein, R., and Marder, J.,** The acid base balance of the rock partridge (*Alectoris Chukur*) exposed to high ambient temperatures, *Comp. Biochem. Physiol.,* 57A, 245, 1977.

62. **Bech, C., Johansen, K., and Maloiy, G. O.,** Ventilation and expired gas composition in the flamingo (*Phoenicopterus ruber*) during normal respiration and panting, *Physiol. Zool.,* 52, 313, 1979.

63. **Murrish, D. E.,** Acid-base balance in three species of Antarctic penguins exposed to thermal stress, *Physiol. Zool.,* 55(2), 137, 1982.

64. **Graf, R.,** Diurnal changes of thermoregulatory functions in pigeons, *Pflügers Arch.,* 386, 173, 1980.

65. **Aschoff, J.,** Der Tagesgang der Körpertemperatur von Vögeln als Funktion des Körpergewichtes, *J. Orn.,* 122, 129, 1981.

66. **Hinds, D. S. and Calder, W. A.,** Tracheal dead space in the respiration of birds, *Evolution,* 25, 429, 1971.

67. **Gleeson, M. and Brackenbury, J. H.,** Ventilation, gaseous exchange and air sac gases during moderate thermal panting in domestic fowl, *Quart. J. Exp. Physiol.,* 68, 591, 1983.

68. **Hales, J. R. S. and Webster, M. E. D.,** Respiratory function during thermal tachypnoea in sheep, *J. Physiol.,* 190, 241, 1967.

69. **Slutsky, A. S., Drazen, J. M., Ingram, R. H., Kamm, R. D., Shapiro, A. H., Fredberg, J. J., Loring, S. H., and Lehr, J.,** Effective pulmonary ventilation with small-volume oscillations at high frequency, *Science,* 209, 609, 1980.

70. **Banzett, R. B. and Lehr, J. L.,** Gas exchange during high-frequency ventilation of the chicken, *J. Appl. Physiol.: Respirat. Environ. Exercise Physiol.,* 53(6), 1418, 1982.

71. **Bretz, W. L. and Schmidt-Nielsen, K.,** Bird respiration: flow patterns in the duck lung, *J. Exp. Biol.,* 54, 103, 1971.

72. **Barnas, G. M., Banzett, R. B., Jones, J. H., Butler, J., and Lehr, J. L.,** Direct test of aerodynamic valving in the avian lung, *Fed. Proc.,* 44, 1384, 1985.

73. **Kanematsu, S., Kii, M., Sonada, T., and Kato, Y.,** Effects of hypothalamic lesions on body temperature in the chicken, *Jpn. J. Vet. Sci.,* 29, 95, 1967.

74. **Lepkovsky, S., Snapir, N., and Furuta, F.,** Temperature regulation and appetitive behaviour in chickens with hypothalamic lesions, *Physiol. Behav.,* 3, 911, 1968.

75. **Richards, S. A. and Avery, P.,** Central nervous mechanisms regulating thermal panting, in *Respiratory Function in Birds, Adult and Embryonic,* Piiper, J., Ed., Springer-Verlag, Berlin, 1978, 196.

76. **Richards, S. A.,** Brain stem control of polypnoea in the chicken and pigeon, *Respir. Physiol.,* 11, 315, 1971.

77. **Richards, S. A.,** Thermal homeostasis in birds, in *Avian Physiology,* Peaker, M., Ed., Academic Press, New York, 1975, 65.

78. **Rautenberg, W.,** Die Bedeutung der zentralnervösen Thermosensitivität für die Temperaturregulation der Taube, *Z. Vgl. Physiol.,* 62, 235, 1969.

79. **Rautenberg, W., Necker, R., and May, B.,** Thermoregulatory responses of the pigeon to changes of the brain and spinal cord temperature, *Pflügers Arch.,* 338, 31, 1972.

80. **Rautenberg, W., May, B., Necker, R., and Rosner, G.,** Control of panting by thermosensitive spinal neurons in birds, in *Respiratory Function in Birds, Adult and Embryonic,* Piiper, J., Ed., Springer-Verlag, Berlin, 1978, 204.

81. **Rautenberg, W.,** Thermoregulation, in *Physiology and Behaviour of the Pigeon,* Abs, M., Ed., Academic Press, New York, 1983, chap. 8.

82. **Richards, S. A.,** The significance of changes in the temperature of the skin and body core of the chicken in the regulation of heat loss, *J. Physiol. (London),* 216, 1, 1971.

83. **Rautenberg, W.,** The influence of the skin temperature on the thermoregulatory system of pigeons, *J. Physiol. (Paris),* 63, 396, 1971.

84. **Hiestand, W. A. and Randall, W. C.,** Influence of proprioceptive vagal afferents on panting and accessory panting movements in mammals and birds, *Am. J. Physiol.,* 138, 12, 1942.

85. **Richards, S. A.,** Vagal control of thermal panting in mammals and birds, *J. Physiol. (London),* 199, 89, 1968.

86. **Barnas, G. M., Estavillo, J. A., Mather, F. B., and Burger, R. E.,** The effect of CO_2 and temperature on respiratory movements in the chicken, *Respir. Physiol.,* 43, 315, 1981.

87. **Barnas, G. M. and Burger, R. E.,** Interaction of temperature with extra- and intrapulmonary chemoreceptor control of ventilatory movements in the awake chicken, *Respir. Physiol.,* 54, 223, 1983.

88. **Brackenbury, J. H.,** Experimentally induced antagonism of chemical and thermal reflexes in the respiratory system of fully conscious chickens, *Respir. Physiol.,* 34, 377, 1978.

89. **Barnas, G. M., Mückenhoff, K., and Scheid, P.,** unpublished observation, 1984.

90. **Brackenbury, J. H. and Gleeson, M.,** Effects of P_{CO_2} on respiratory pattern during thermal and exercise hyperventilation in domestic fowl, *Respir. Physiol.,* 54, 109, 1983.

91. **Dawson, W. R. and Hudson, J. W.,** Birds, in *Comparative Physiology of Thermoregulation,* Vol. 1, Whittow, G. C., Ed., Academic Press, New York, 1970, 223.

92. **Rautenberg, W.,** Temperature regulation in cold environment, in *Acta 17. Congr. Int. Ornithol.,* Nönring, R., Ed., Verlag der Deutschen Ornithologen Gesellschaft, Berlin, 1980.

93. **Hemingway, A.,** Shivering, *Physiol. Rev.,* 43, 397, 1963.

94. **Rautenberg, W.,** Untersuchungen zur Temperaturregulation wärme- und kälteaklimatisierter Tauben, *Z. Vl. Physiol.,* 62, 221, 1969.

95. **Janský, L.,** Non-shivering thermogenesis and its thermoregulatory significance, *Biol. Rev.,* 48, 85, 1973.

96. **Simon, E.,** Temperature regulation: the spinal cord as a site of extrahypothalamic thermoregulation functions, *Rev. Physiol. Biochem. Pharmacol.,* 71, 1, 1974.

97. **Necker, R.,** Temperature-sensitive ascending neurons in the spinal cord of pigeons, *Pflügers Arch.,* 353, 275, 1975.

98. **Necker, R.,** Thermoreception and temperature regulation in homeothermic vertebrates, in *Sensory Physiology 2,* Autrum, H., Ottoson, D., Perl, E., and Schmidt, R. F., Eds., Springer-Verlag, Berlin, 1981.

99. **Necker, R. and Rautenberg, W.,** Effect of spinal deafferentation on temperature regulation and spinal thermosensitivity in pigeons, *Pflügers Arch.,* 360, 287, 1975.

100. **Barnas, G. and Rautenberg, W.,** Respiratory responses to shivering produced by external and central cooling in the pigeon, *Pflügers Arch.,* 401, 228, 1984.

101. **Bouverot, P., Hildwein, G., and Oulhen, P.,** Ventilatory and circulatory O_2 convection at 4000 m in pigeon at neutral or cold temperature, *Respir. Physiol.,* 28, 371, 1976.

102. **Bernstein, M. H. and Schmidt-Nielsen, K.,** Ventilation and oxygen extraction in the crow, *Respir. Physiol.,* 21, 393, 1974.

103. **Bech, C., Johansen, K., Brent, R., and Nicol, S.,** Ventilatory and circulatory changes during cold exposure in the pekin duck *(Anas platyrhynchos), Respir. Physiol.,* 57, 103, 1984.

104. **Brent, R., Rasmussen, J. G., Bech, C., and Martini, S.,** Temperature dependence of ventilation and O_2-extraction in the kittiwake, *Rissa tridactyla, Experientia,* 39, 1092, 1983.

105. **Brent, R., Federsen, P. F., Bech, C., and Johansen, K.,** Lung ventilation and temperature regulation in the European coot *(Fulica Atra), Physiol. Zool.,* 57, 19, 1984.

106. **Johansen, K. and Bech, C.,** Heat conservation during cold exposure in birds (vasomotor and respiratory implications), *Polar Res.,* 1, 259, 1983.

107. **DiMarco, A. F., Romaniuk, J. R., von Euler, C., and Yamamoto, Y.,** Immediate changes in ventilation and respiratory pattern associated with onset and cessation of locomotion in the cat, *J. Physiol. (London),* 343, 1, 1983.

108. **Barnas, G., Nomoto, S., and Rautenberg, W.,** Cardiovascular and bloods gas responses to shivering produced by external and central cooling in the pigeon, *Pflügers Arch.,* 401, 223, 1984.

109. **Bech, C. and Rautenberg, W.,** unpublished observations, 1984.

Index

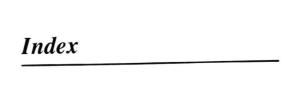

INDEX

Q

R